Medicine as a Human Science

Norelle Lickiss

Medicine as a Human Science

Edited by Jean Curthoys

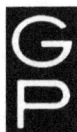

GP

Medicine as a Human Science
ISBN 978 1 76109 384 5
Copyright © text Norelle Lickiss 2022

First published 2022 by
GINNINDERRA PRESS
PO Box 3461 Port Adelaide 5015
www.ginninderrapress.com.au

Contents

A Note from the Editor 7

Part One

Introduction: Medicine is a Human Science 11

1   The Human Experience of Illness 21

2   On the Shape of Human Suffering 38

3   On the Kindness of Strangers 52

Part Two

4   Diagnosis and Prognosis 65

Part Three

5   Living in the Decade of the Dying 81

6   After the Decade for Dying, What Now? 89

Postscript

7   The Evolution of the Ecological Concept of a Person 101

Notes 110

Bibliography 117

A Note from the Editor

Dr Norelle Lickiss has had a distinguished career as a medical clinician and researcher. She has many publications in medical journals and edited books, but the ideas presented here are of a different order in that they concern the very nature of medical practice. These are philosophical reflections, both in the ancient sense of philosophy as 'the love of wisdom' and in the way they draw on the work of professional philosophers. At the same time, they are about medicine as science, these two strands coming together in Norelle's central thesis that medicine is a human science. These ideas have been developed, worked over and refined over six decades but have seen the light of day infrequently, in the occasional address or lecture. This has been in spite of repeated requests from Norelle's colleagues that she write them up for publication, making them accessible to a wider audience.

I have been privileged, then, to be allowed to edit some mountains of Norelle's papers to produce this book. I have selected those which I think best illuminate the conception of medicine as a human science. To some extent I have also tightened up the prose, since much of what I received was in draft form. Since I am a philosopher, not a medico, by training this means that, unfortunately, much of Norelle's distinctive voice, as expressed in the rhythm of her prose, has been lost and replaced by my own rather more prosaic tone. It also means that any mistakes are almost surely mine.

My aim has been to highlight the main ideas which, I believe, are of no small significance for both philosophy and medicine. The bringing of philosophy to medicine in effect outlines philosophical foundations for the latter, while her plea to philosophers to take seriously the experience of doctors is yet another reminder that philosophy can too easily lose its grounding in the real world of lived experience. Doctors, in relating to patients, have a very special experience of human relationships, one which can deepen our understanding of the nature of the human person. The idea of medicine as a human science centres on that understanding. This is something more than 'person-centred medicine' in the way that notion is now popularly used. As Norelle says, if we are to talk of 'person-centred' medicine, we have to have a deeper understanding of just what a person is and the current talk of the person as an autonomous, decision-making agent can be insufficient when treating the ill. It is in enlarging our conception of 'the person' that medicine, conducted as a human science, can make its distinctive contribution to philosophy, to medicine and more widely to the culture at large.

Part One

Introduction

Medicine is a Human Science

The task of medical practitioners – indeed, our privilege – is to be with people in their illness. In this, we have a responsibility to embody the humane, the authentically human. By being with others as *they* experience challenging, often life-limiting situations, the experience and understanding we acquire is unique. Doctors are applied scientists but we also try to act beneficently, truly respecting each person we encounter, whether rich or poor, criminal or law-abiding, friendly combatant or so-called enemy. We make no distinctions save on severity of need. Some of us, like our colleagues in *Médecins Sans Frontières,* pursue this calling even at the cost of our lives. For most of us, the challenges are less dramatic but even so, in our professional daily life, they are ever present.

We rarely speak of the view of humanity which impels us. Yet because of our particular insights into human beings, we could, if we dared, make a distinctive contribution, not only to medical science, but also to more general, philosophical thought. We could be part of the shaping of a new humanism – a humanist understanding for our time. In his allegorical novel *The Plague*, it is to the doctor (Rieux) that Camus attributes the conviction that there is more good to admire in people than there is evil to despise, and certainly that is something that we doctors do know. But we know more than that and the understanding of human beings which we acquire in our work expands and deepens as the years go on. This book contains the late thoughts of a senior clinician.

Medicine is a human science. This is not a truism but a substantive claim based on an accepted distinction between the natural sciences and the human sciences.[1] It is also a controversial claim because there are many who take it for granted that medicine belongs unequivocally only with the natural sciences – the so-called hard sciences of physics, chemistry, biology and geology. The human sciences are more loosely defined but are commonly thought to contain what are known as the humanities – history, sociology, anthropology, psychology, economics, but also literature and philosophy. Whereas the natural sciences proceed by observation and experiment, the human sciences rely on argument, reflection and introspection (as well as observation) *to interpret the meaningful dimension* of human behaviour. They are distinguished principally by the fact that they incorporate an understanding of the subjective inner world. The debate about where medicine belongs is important because if it is seen primarily to belong to the natural science of biology – which is, of course, an essential component – its very core is lost. Medicine is about humanity – humanity in the form of individual men and women and their communities. More precisely, it is concerned with those impediments to human flourishing which stem from the suboptimal or malfunctioning of the human body. Its aim is, where possible, to remove these impediments.

Now it is philosophy which has explored the nature of human flourishing, seeking to identify both how it is enabled and how it is impeded. When we conceptualise human possibility (which medical practitioners are tacitly doing constantly), we are thinking philosophically. Medicine, then, needs an explicitly philosophic component. If that is absent, if the 'humanness' at the heart of medicine is lost, then the biological science may be seriously misdirected. This 'humanness' of medicine goes deeper than the fact that medicine is about human beings and deeper, even, than the fact that its ideals are to assist human flourishing. The very practice of medicine involves some of the most fundamentally human responses one human being can have to another. I came to this rare insight after a memorable address by legal theorist Professor Desmond Manderson, in which he drew on the thought of the French philosopher Emanuel Levinas, to argue that medical practice is grounded in the necessity to respond to *the call of the other in need.* Manderson's point was that, while any decent man or woman will, where they can, go to the aid of another in need, doctors have such a response as a core requirement of their life.[2] Yes, there are always limits to availability and appropriateness of response, but the fundamental orientation of a medical practitioner should bear the mark of radical availability. Another way of looking at this is to recognise that patients place on doctors an obligation to care which is based on a radical love for mankind.

The ideas advanced here, then, belong broadly to the realm of philosophy. They are a contribution to the development of a philosophical component of medical practice. That said, I need to be very clear that I am not writing *as* a philosopher but simply as a person exploring her personal world and sometimes finding the insights of philosophers illuminating in giving form to my musings as I stumble towards deeper meaning. What these essays are *not* are strictly philosophical engagements with centuries of thought about the human condition. Nor do they belong to what is currently in vogue as intellectual discourse. What they *are*, in part, is an attempt to integrate some of the experience of a long life, lived somewhat in counterpoint, impelled by passion (occasionally misguided) and moulded by the sharing of profound times with thousands of patients. Such deep encounters engage one's mind in concert with one's heart.

*

The human experience of each of us, in its manifold arenas, is a legitimate resource. It is more than a topic to be reflected on and written about as an object of study, although I once did just that.[3] Since then, I have learned that it is experience which not only shapes our response to questions but actually poses them in the first place. And in my experience, my wonderings have oscillated between two questions, occupying the space in between. They are the questions 'Who am I?' and 'What do we mean by "God"?' I am scarcely alone in this, of course. In every age there have been those seeking to explicitly address both these questions, struggling with the conviction, on the one hand, that they, themselves, are the source of their actions and moral judgements, and, on the other, that there is a question about what we might call the 'all that is'. The dilemma goes back as far as Gilgamesh's questioning of the nature and necessity of death and, ever since, it has resurfaced regularly in philosophical and religious thought. In the Hebrew scriptures, Cain questioned the nature of responsibility ('Am I my brother's keeper?'); Buddha questioned the nature and necessity of suffering; Moses, feeling he was being addressed in his encounter with the burning-bush-not-consumed, asked (of God?) 'Who are You?', and so on. Great music and art cry out these questions which seem to be the stuff of our striving. Perhaps every person lives their life between these two questions, the tension between which manifests in human conflict whether as internal conflict in individuals, philosophical conflict between individuals, or military conflict when wars are fought over the nature or existence of God. It is my belief that the specific experience of medical practitioners dealing with the ill and the dying can help bridge the gap between the earthly 'I' and the seemingly transcendent 'G' (however the latter is understood).

A new humanism

Above all, it is our patients who are our teachers. It is they who educate us, in the full and original sense of that word, which derives from both the Latin *educere* (to lead) and *educare* (to nourish). So we could say that 'to educate' is to lead us out from where we are to a new place, sustaining us as we make the journey. Patient after patient challenges us. In the first instance, of course, the challenge is to understand their ailment in order to alleviate it. But our responsibility to be humane provides us with other challenges. One of them is to identify the wellsprings of a courage and resilience in the face of what we, ourselves, may not be able to bear. Seemingly small things, like an amulet held fast, or an icon above the bed, may indicate that our patients might live, often then to die, in a world quite alien to the one we highly educated professionals mostly inhabit.[4] Finally, we learn, perhaps initially to our surprise, that our patients nourish, nurture and care for us.

In these essays, references will be made to recent writers who are worth noting because of the way they weave together the above and other related strands of thoughts: Jacob Needleman, Thomasine Kushner, Karen Armstrong and John Hick, to mention some of them.

The Humanist Frame (edited by Julian Huxley) interested me in the early years of my professional career and still provides an appropriate point of departure.[5] Huxley's preface contains the following:

> This book is an attempt to present Humanism as a comprehensive system of ideas. It is no sudden venture, but the natural outcome of a long process of gestation and development, begun more than half a century ago, in an attempt to reconcile or integrate various aspects of my life – my biological training, my twin loves of nature and poetry, my wrestlings with the problems of morality and belief…

Later, Huxley asserts his interest in 'the emergence of a new comprehensive pattern or system of ideas, beliefs and guiding principles which are of general validity for the entire human community'. It was this insistence on the emergence of a new humanism, combined with his attempt to reconcile his scientific training with philosophical exploration, which moved me to begin my own search to contribute to humanist thought. Huxley's words were penned in the midst of the 'terrible beauty'[6] of the twentieth century, but since then there have been massive shifts in the intellectual climate, especially since the close of that century. We now live in an ocean of information, guests, as it were, at an immeasurably gigantic smorgasbord in cyberspace, most information we seek available at our fingertips. We drown in a surfeit of facts. At the same time, people are becoming increasingly aware that information alone is not understanding and that understanding is not, in itself, wisdom – for as well as understanding, wisdom requires the exercise of right judgement. The conflict between a virtual oversupply of information on the one hand and understanding and wisdom on the other is particularly clear in medical practice, where reliance on the quantitative has somewhat displaced the inherently subjective 'right judgment'.[7] Our intellectual climate is now critically dependent on cyberspace, the possible collapse of which has the potential to cripple affluent nations. It is in this new radically new and unprecedented climate that any new 'comprehensive pattern or system of ideas, beliefs and guiding principles' will be formed.

If too much information and a reliance on the quantitative erodes deeper understanding, there are countervailing tendencies in a growing appreciation of human diversity, a greater awareness of poverty/hunger/disease, deeper understanding of strivings for liberty and human rights and of their repression by dictators, both secular and religious. In short, there is an ongoing reappraisal of history – part of a process of disillusionment with ideas and institutions hitherto assumed to be worthy of trust and praise. Moreover – and of particular significance to the medical profession – is the maturing realisation that the Nazi holocaust was not just another terrible violent event but a hiatus in human history, a final crashing down of the dreams of the enlightenment in an apparently civilised nation with a glorious intellectual history.[8] The respect once accorded to the German academic medical tradition proved to be badly misplaced with the realisation of the unspeakable failure of Nazi doctors to exercise basic morality. Henry Sigerist, who devoted his life to studying the history of medicine, pointed out that medical practice occurs in a historical context, mirroring the ideas and values of that context. Maybe, then, we can think of our medical practice as a canary in a coal mine, alerting observers to hazardous currents in the way that the moral collapse of Nazi doctors revealed the realities of their context. But if the actions and ideas of doctors take their cue from the world in which we are embedded, then there surely needs to be an instinct, too, for independent thought, maybe even an intellectual rebellion, honed by profound study and reflection. We should incorporate, not forget, the fundamental insights of the wisest forebears in the traditions which we embody.

However, the residues of wisdom which we have are in written words and even the intelligentsia refer to these much less frequently than they did in earlier times and they are rarely found in the hands of those in power. Seldom are they pondered and reflected upon – there is no time for that. Time is taken up by trivia, inordinate recording of data and compliance with pointless regulations. Writers themselves have little time to read the carefully crafted words of other writers. The potential of our intrinsic human freedom may be fading. The countervailing tendency depends on those who emerge in every generation and are able to embody deep human truths despite, or because of, the dark times in which they live.

Our times are not Huxley's times and, in any case, we cannot be as confident as he was that we are at any kind of threshold. That will only be known at a distance, not from within the turbulence. All we can know is that in our time and place, too, we need to be wholly present, to create (whether in art, or words, or life) and to care for each other and the earth in dignity. For, as a recently deceased philosopher wrote,

> Without dignity our lives are only blinks of duration. But if we manage to lead a good life well, we create something more. We write a subscript to our mortality. We make our lives tiny diamonds in the cosmic sands.[9]

The person

Many decades ago, the philosopher Jacob Needleman pointed to what he saw as a damaging blind spot in medical practice: 'What medicine lacks', he wrote, 'is any fundamental notion of the nature of man and any remotely adequate understanding of that to which we refer as a person.'[10] I was a young doctor when I read these words. At the time, I naturally assumed that I understood what a person was. Of course I knew! Only as the decades rolled on and I reflected on the regularity with which patients complain that they wanted to be treated like a person, did I begin to realise what Needleman meant. And it was then that I started to develop the following concept of a person.

Needleman's point accompanies Mandelson's, for if our basic commitment is to the call of the other, it is not to the other as the bearer of a diseased or damaged body, but to the other as person (with diseased or damaged body). The absence of a concept of a person is an absence at the core of medicine's self-understanding. To put it differently, if medicine is a human science, it requires a conception of a person – its philosophical component will centre on developing that conception. Without an understanding of personhood, it will shrink to an applied biological science.

The experience of many years has made me increasingly aware that humanity is complex. As a species, our complexity manifests in diversity, that is, in differences in our physicality, in the way we think, in our aspirations and in what we do. Underlying that diversity is the complexity of a single human being, and it is that which became my focus. Its general features started to become clear to me in the course of my first serious research ,which was into aspects of indigenous health. I realised that to understand a person as a person, one has to consider their current environment, their personal history (as they remember/interpret it) and the biological and cultural inheritance upon which they have been built. But the overarching and fundamental insight was that these relationships are not added to a person but actually constitute a person.

This relational concept of a person is ontological in that it concerns the kind of being a person is. And so 'Who am I?', one of my two fundamental questions, received a preliminary answer at that ontological level: 'I am a fragile web of relationships.' This conception fits well with – indeed, it underpins – the influential view of suffering[11] as a sense of impending personal disintegration, a sense of being about to go to pieces.

The understanding of a person as constituted by their relations became the basis of further thinking and clinical work. In subsequent decades, it was developed around a number of additional themes. An important one concerned the critical significance of hope – for one of the most searching and sometimes painful questions to ask a very ill patient is 'What do you hope for now?' I came to understand hope as a kind of dynamic vector capable of preventing the 'fragile web' of a person from locking in on itself and becoming a closed system.

Another theme, this one broaching my second fundamental question about God, departed from the realisation that the system of relations coheres until whatever held it together passes away at death. The relations which constitute a person call for a principle of integration: I think that is what spirit is. Weakening or cleavage of even one of these constitutive relations may be the trigger for suffering as defined by Cassell as a sense of impending personal disintegration.[11] In common parlance, we may say that loss of my child/spouse/house/land/books/ dignity/culture and so on 'broke my spirit'. (This is a conception which could ground a profound view of spiritual care.) For every person must have a mythology energising their life, and a frame of some sort for such a complexus.

Each of us needs some ritual in the frame of our lives, and indeed some myths to live by. For some, these take a religious form. It may be timely to assert that radical humanism not only does not exclude religion but may include it as a human construction expressing several constitutive relations, notably with other persons in one's present and past, with some things perceived as sacred, and with the whole of reality.

Almost all the essays in this book develop this relational concept of a person as I seek to apply and expand within the specifically human dimensions of medical practice. The first essay, about the human experience of illness, illustrates what it means to understand medicine as a human science rather than as an exclusively natural science. There are essays of a more general philosophical nature which explore, amongst other themes, the nature of human suffering, medical care, human dignity and the kindness of strangers. Other essays apply these understandings to the specific problems of diagnosis, prognosis, clinical decision-making and a doctor's role in society. There is some repetition and overlap between the chapters, which are also intended to be read as independent essays, although many will also refer back to other chapters.

All are intended as a contribution to the understanding and development of medicine as a human science.

1

The Human Experience of Illness

Illness is the night side of life, a more onerous citizenship. Everyone who is born holds dual citizenship, in the kingdom of the well and in the kingdom of the sick. Although we all prefer to use only the good passport, sooner or later each of us is obliged, at least for a spell, to identify ourselves as citizens of that other place. (Susan Sontag)[1]

What is illness? Illness is a personal, not a biological, condition.. It is usually defined as a deviation from health, adequate definitions of which also go beyond the hard scientific medical facts. Understanding that, Johannes Bircher defines health as 'a state of well-being characterised by a physical, mental and social potential, which satisfies the demands of a life commensurate with age, culture and personal responsibility'.[2] The World Health Organisation echoes these notions. Illness, then, is contrasted with disease, which term is mainly used to refer to an objectively verifiable disturbance of bodily structure or function. A person may or may not be conscious of their disease. Illness, on the other hand, involves subjective awareness of a state deviating from an individual's normal state of well-being. Illness is intrinsically experiential and may or may not be easy to describe. Disease may be manifest in imaging, in biochemical studies, in histopathology and so on, but illness is not so demonstrable and, although its behavioural concomitants may be observable, the illness itself is not.

Further, illness may occur without demonstrable disease, either because the disease cannot be identified, or because the illness is of a predominantly psychological nature. Conversely, disease may be present without illness. (For example, rising levels of tumour markers herald recurrence of symptomless ovarian cancer.) In such cases, though, illness may appear later in the form of severe anxiety or depression, or sometimes just as a result of such information being conveyed. A cancer survivor may go to a follow-up appointment feeling well but leave the consulting room a citizen of the kingdom of the ill.

Illness, then, is a manifestation of the human condition and so may be studied through any one of the prisms of history, art, literature, philosophy, sociology, psychology, theology, economics or political science – any of the prisms, that is, which refract the light impinging on the human intellect. The study of disease relates medical science to the natural sciences. The experience of illness is not marginal to the human condition, nor an aberrant optional extra at the edge of human affairs – it is central. Illness is core business for a human person and almost always embedded in the pattern of a life.[3] It is because it is the study of illness as well as disease that medicine is a human science.[4]

Towards an adequate view of person

If illness is an intensely personal, subjective reality, then medical practice requires an adequate concept of a person.[5] It is some decades ago that Jacob Needleman pointed out medicine's lack of any adequate understanding of the nature of man or of what we refer to as a person. That lack has yet to be filled and in the following I propose the broad outlines of how this might be done, mindful that the framework I present must be sufficiently simple to be held as part of the 'furniture of the mind'.[6]

Defining a person is an age-old problem, one which before modern times was addressed mostly within religious or spiritual traditions. Sacred writings issued what remain as wise counsel about the human condition, often doing so in the shape of powerful myths embodying deep truths. In addition, vast tomes of a more philosophical or theological nature about the nature of man, the meaning of man, images of man and so forth have been produced in both East and West. All that is relevant here. However, what is needed to underpin contemporary clinical practice, while in no way eschewing these religious traditions, has to relate to our secular world. Philosophical anthropology is the branch of philosophy which attempts to understand the person or, otherwise put, the human condition. It is a pursuit broad enough to encompass insights from both religious and humanist traditions without being confined to either. In short, what contemporary medicine lacks is a philosophical anthropology and that is what the following will attempt to sketch.

Many of the medical practitioners, students and other health care professionals to whom my thoughts are specifically addressed will lack philosophical training but I believe they will find the concepts accessible simply in virtue of the fact that they are, themselves, immersed in the human condition. Moreover, they are immersed in a particularly intense way, for as well as living their lives as individual human persons, they are in the midst of others who need their skills and judgement, many of whom will be in extreme distress. There has to be a two-way dynamic in developing medicine as a human science. If medical clinical practice needs a philosophical anthropology, conversely philosophical anthropology needs to extend to an understanding of the specific experiences that the medical clinician can describe. To understand the human condition, we need to understand it in both illness and in health. If the doctors need the philosophers, the philosophers equally need to listen to the doctors.

*

There is a simple framework I have found to be useful in clinical teaching. It is, I think, sufficiently straightforward to function as 'furniture of the mind'. I have labelled it an 'ecological view of a person' since it centres on the idea of a person as an intrinsically relational concept – *intrinsically* relational, for the idea is not just that a person has relations with others and with the world but that s/he is *constituted* as an individual person by these relations. Its importance to clinical practice is that it emphasises what is imperative for both patients and carers (lay or professional) to keep in mind when the patient's distress is evident, for it is then that these constitutive relations are most significant.

In the first instance, these relations are identified as those with the current environment. Here they amount to a continuous and dialectical interaction between person and object (other people, things or places). The philosopher Charles Taylor expressed it well: '[personal identity] is defined by the commitments and identifications which provide the frame or the horizon' and 'I am a self only in relation to certain inter-locutors: in relation to those conversation partners who were essential to my achieving self definition.' For Taylor, a self exists only within 'webs of interlocution'. As to why these 'webs of interlocution' are so fundamental,

> To ask what a person is, in abstraction, from his or her self-inter-pretations, is to ask a fundamentally misguided question, one to which there couldn't, in principle, be an answer... We are only selves insofar as we move in a certain space of questions, as we seek and find an orientation to the good.[7]

In sum, a person is their self-understanding, but that understanding is gained only in dialogue with the people and objects which thereby become part of the person.

There is more: a person is not only in relation with their present life-situation but also with their personal past. For medical staff, the essential historicity of a person, elucidated so profoundly by Taylor, is a practical consideration. It is not only the facts of the past (medical, so-cial, psychological) which are pertinent, for the manner in which the patient understands, incorporates and interprets that past, is equally relevant, if not more so. For the clinician seeking to restore, rehabilitate, or to continue to care for a patient, neglect of the patient's historicity may inhibit the possibility of relieving suffering. Never is this more im-portant than in situations of predictable deterioration, or in those of approaching death.

The inheritance of a person can be seen as the platform and scaffold-ing on which, and within which, one's self-interpretation is constructed.

In effect, it is one's personal history, since self-interpretation is essentially historical. That inheritance has two dimensions: biological and cultural. The biological consists in the genetic influence on disease, although it can also have much of personal or social significance; the cultural is related to ethnicity, occupation, social circumstance or religious tradition and is the atmosphere which a person breathes from cradle to grave. The cultural will influence both what happens and the interpretation of what happens; it will give shape to the self and to emotional response, whether it be anxiety, fear, hope or despair.

Walt Whitman said all this, very succinctly, in the mid-nineteenth century: 'I am not contained between my hat and my boots.'[8] Likewise, Henry James, in the late nineteenth century:

a man's 'me' is the sum total of all that he can call his, not only his body and his mind, but his clothes and his house, his wife and his children, his ancestors and his friends, his reputation and his works, his lands and horses, his yacht and his bank account.[9]

And Ernest Becker, whose 1973 book *Denial of Death* influenced a whole generation, used his colourful imagination to describe the relations which make us what we are:

You get a good feeling for what the self 'looks like' if you imagine the person to be a cylinder with a hollow inside, in which is lodged his self. Out of this cylinder the self overflows and extends into the surroundings, as a kind of huge amoeba, pushing its pseudopodia to a wife, a car, a flag, a crushed flower in a secret book. The picture you get is of a huge invisible amoeba spread out over the landscape, with boundaries very far from its own centre or home base. Tear and burn the flag, find and destroy the flower in the book, and the amoeba screams with soul-searing pain.[10]

But there is more to the concept of a person and it is here that medical practice has something specific to offer philosophical anthropology. The medical professional needs to be especially attuned to the contrast between hope and despair and the possibility that the latter might trap the person within a closed system. In those cases, hope can be a means of transcendence, a transcendence which then becomes part of the core reality of a person. Nowhere is this more crucial than in the last phase of life when the task is to move towards a sense of the wholeness of life, rooted in faith in 'that which will not fail' – such things as the fidelity of others, or one's own enduring worth. If hope fails, the outcome can be despair, so clinicians need to be aware of the tragic consequences of falsely oriented hope. The complexity of the relationships (not only those of family) which contain, restrain and support, and through which the patient functions as a person, needs to be appreciated, even if a busy physician or nurse gains only a glimmering.

In the foregoing, the attempt has been to avoid those aspects of the Western framework which are not applicable in other cultural contexts, which is not to say that cultural differences are not relevant. Humanity is one, and some matters are universal. There may be cultural disagreements on specifics, for example on the kind of relations with others which constitute the person, or on the degree and nature of attachment to place. But Becker's rather dramatic portrayal of the extended self rings true everywhere in the kingdom of the ill, even if there is no wife, car or flag – just the crushed flower of a precious memory. Illness everywhere has the potential to manifest in soul-searing pain by touching unexpected aspects of the self.

Personal development

A person is an intrinsically relational reality and also a dynamic reality, ever-changing, often imperceptibly. Development is not merely structural (in terms of cell turnover and so on) for it occurs within the functioning whole – the self is constantly being fashioned and refashioned. In order to facilitate rather than inhibit personal growth, it is essential for a clinician without formal training in psychology or psychiatry to have some grasp of the way persons develop, especially during life crises. Volumes have been written about this[11] – indeed, the discipline of developmental psychology is devoted to the subject. But once again, a manageable schema is needed by the practising clinician to make sense of the tapestry of phenomena manifesting personal change and development as it occurs in the everyday stuff of clinical practice. The following summary of the ideas of Erik Erikson, which are relatively inaccessible in the original, might help supply that need. They are ideas which have stood the test of time.[12]

In essence, Erikson saw human growth as emerging from the negotiation of developmental tasks by way of the resolution of crises. The human being, he maintained, is continually facing options, each life stage being characterised by choices specific to it and which, while continuing throughout life, come to a point of ascendancy in that stage. For example, the choice in infancy is between trust and distrust, the favourable outcome being an attitude of basic trust. In the toddler years, the choice is between autonomy and fear of decision-making, and the outcome will be influenced by that of the previous stage. Further choices are faced in subsequent life stages.

Where the life process is characterised by the embracing of favourable options, the personality becomes characterised by trust, reasonable autonomy, initiative, capacity for effort and a sense of identity, that is, a sense of being oneself, with a willingness to share oneself. There is, in those cases, a capacity for intimate personal relationships (to lose and find oneself in another) instead of isolation; fruitfulness as opposed to stagnation and, finally, a sense of the integrity or wholeness of life, the alternative being despair. The negotiations of these developmental tasks involve personal relationships and the whole spectrum of human communication, both in the present, and between the past and present. In the course of such communication, life cycles, as Erikson called them, are interlocked, cog-wheeled as it were, welding together the human community into a matrix, in a continuous process or movement.

This analysis of personal growth contains a profound understanding of the developmental task of the elderly and of those of any age approaching death. That task he conceived as the final stage in the development of a sense of wholeness, of integrity.

Only he who in some way has taken care of things and people and has adapted himself to the triumphs and disappointments of being, by necessity, the originator of others and the generator of things and ideas – only he may gradually grow the fruit of the seven stages. I know no better word for it than integrity… It is the acceptance of one's own and only life cycle and of the people who have become significant to it as something that had to be…an acceptance of the fact that one's life is one's own responsibility. It is a sense of comradeship with men and women of distant times and of different pursuits, who have created orders and objects and sayings conveying human dignity and love.[13]

But he noted further,

…the lack or loss of this accrued ego integration is signified by despair and an often unconscious fear of death: the one and only life cycle is not accepted as the ultimate of life. Despair expresses the fear that the time is short, too short for the attempt to start another life and to try out alternative roads to integrity. Such a despair is often hidden behind a show of disgust, a misanthropy, or a chronic contemptuous displeasure with (where not allied with constructive ideas and life of co-operation) only signify the individual's contempt of himself.[14]

The human responses to these crises are the stuff of opera, movies, novels and plays. Challenges of effort, of intimacy, of creativity, of generativity, of loss, of failure, of guilt, of facing dissolution – these are the landmarks of human life, not all present in all lives (except inchoately) but explicit in most. Any physician who has cared for dying children or adolescents knows that chronological age is not what defines whether or not a named developmental challenge is discernible. The sequence of the stages described may be telescoped into a few years: the old, or even simply the adult, have no monopoly of the whole.

Erikson has been quoted at length because his lengthier writings are relatively inaccessible, while the tasks he describes need to be understood by those in contact with patients undergoing a life crisis. Nowhere is this understanding more crucial than with those approaching death, who may well vacillate between wholeness and despair and who need to be supported gently. They may long to, and need to, express their internal states, explore the threat of despair and, through dialogue with significant others, they may reach out again towards wholeness. If it is the task of each person to explore the limits of their own possibilities, it is surely the task of the doctor to free a very ill patient, where they can, from obstacles (like pain) to such an exploration. Palliative medicine is concerned with the facilitation of free being, with liberation.

Erikson's sensitive portrayal of the developmental task of the final phase of life throws fresh light on my earlier emphasis on the clinician's role in sustaining and helping to reconstruct hope. If the alternatives are between wholeness and despair, then hope becomes a precondition for wholeness. No person should die in despair and so the clinician should surely assist the patient to centre hope, not on what will in the end probably fail (for example, the tenth line chemotherapy, radiotherapy, surgery) but in what will not fail. The clinician must be committed, not only to the control of pain, but to the patient as a unique, irreplaceable subject of existence. These matters call for much reflection if we are not to add to the despair of those dying, especially those now dying in high-tech contexts.

It is significant that, for Erikson, the final sense of the wholeness of life is an acceptance of one's place, and time, and oneself. The last phase of life, so understood, is an opportunity for growth towards that wholeness occurring (as in a pot plant) from within, but influenced (as it is in the pot plant) by context.

The seasons of illness

Fitzhugh Mullan was a physician and cancer survivor. The experience of the latter, in combination with his expertise, inspired him to formulate the concept of 'the seasons of survival', further specified as the seasons of acute survival, extended survival and permanent survival.[15] His belief was that an appreciation of these seasons would help both patients and health professionals to develop better strategies. Following his call for more research into the subject, attention has been drawn to liminality, a condition which had been recognised in other contexts such as chronic pain.[16] Liminality is, in effect, the phenomenon discussed by Stonequist in his classic study of 'the marginal man', the person who is 'uneasily poised in psychological uncertainty between two (or more) social worlds, reflecting in his soul the discords and harmonies, repulsions and attractions of these worlds, one of which is "dominant" over the other'.[17] Stonequist was concerned with marginality due to ethnicity, but the general idea can be equally applied to the two worlds of the 'kingdom of the well' and the 'kingdom of the sick'. The seasons of survival, it could be said, are characterised by liminality, an existence in both these worlds, necessarily in tension with each other.

This concept of seasons, however, need not be confined to the phase of survival and could well be used in relation to the different phases of illness, all of which might be experienced by one person in the course of one disease, whether or not it proves fatal. While disease has long been recognised to have definable phases, to date, illness has not.[18]

Each season of illness, as the experiential dimension of a disease, has definable though variable features and challenges. The following seasons may be delineated: (i) the experience of diagnosis; (ii) treatment; (iii) surveillance; (iv) favourable response; (v) non-response; (v) relapse; (vi) further surveillance; (vii) progression; and (viii) approaching death.[19] Each phase may include many perils – symptoms, uncertainty, ambiguity, delay, difficulties in decision making, loss of many kinds, approaching death.[20] (The experience of liminality may also be mirrored in at least some seasons of their illness, although, as yet, that is only a hypothesis.)

The facing of death, clearly one of the seasons of illness, has been described in literature. For example, Tolstoy's *The Death of Ivan Ilyich* is, for doctors, a disturbing literary icon. Medical texts need to be supplemented by such literature from the humanities because no empirical medical research can capture the entirety of the experience. Then again, no more can philosophers, poets, theologians, or the sacred writings of all peoples. Some uncertainties are at the core of human experience, and the human experience of facing death, though in some measure illuminated, will always belong to the 'riddling essence' of human existence.

Palliative care and illness

There is much written on the definable side-effects of anti-cancer treatments such as surgery, chemotherapy and radiotherapy. Mostly, though, attention has been focused on the improvement of techniques and symptom management, to provide both better and more economical treatment.[21] However, the core competence of palliative medicine practitioners involves more than symptom relief, for it includes support for patients and their families and the clarification of goals for all concerned (immortality not one of them). In short, it is palliative practitioners who deal with both illness and disease, and their services should be available in parallel with all treatment programs in potentially lethal conditions. The more radical the treatment, the more vital are the skills of palliative care personnel. The achievement of this may require a seismic cultural shift in the relationship between specialist palliative care services and oncology and associated medical services, and therefore also in health administration and insurance circles. Only reliable palliative care can bring the benefits of contemporary treatments to patients in such a way that, after the treatment phase, they do not feel that they resemble a battlefield. It is the responsibility of the health care system to assist patients as the seasons of illness unfold, and then with either survival or death.

One practical issue as oncology practice goes global is the irresponsibility of introducing potentially toxic or hazardous anti-cancer treatments into contexts where there is not equal competence in symptom relief and surveillance and in provision of personal and family support. It can be further argued that, in any culture or circumstances, when decisions are being made concerning the treatment options of a very ill patient (for example, whether or not to try further chemotherapy with the goal of trying to prolong life) a carer impact statement is needed because some options will increase the burden on carers. This is not to say that a careful consideration of the patient's wishes is not the prime concern. It would be best if advance care planning were instituted as soon as the illness appeared to be potentially fatal so the patient's wishes were known well in advance, rather than at the point where control of the disease is failing. These matters require urgent discussion and research. The experience of illness impacts on the whole personal field and most especially on carers. The personal is relational.

Emotions

Emotions are respectable. In fact, they are essential! In her discussion of emotional intelligence, Nussbaum stresses from the outset that it is emotions which shape the landscape of our mental and social lives and which, borrowing from Proust, she describes as 'geological upheavals of thought'.[22] These upheavals are common in illness and the thoughts causing them are often due to new information about, or heightened awareness of, one's condition. Such emotional outbreaks need to be understood as manifestations of underlying tensions, not as negative features of personalities.[23] That kind of understanding is one of the aims of the field of psycho-oncology, which has developed as both a clinical and a theoretical discipline, the latter incorporating the insights of psychology and psychiatry.

The relational view of a person provides a useful framework for integrating many of the factors which influence the emotional response of patients in all the seasons of illness of a life threatening disease. These seasons include the particularities of the disease along with the many personal factors identified in that framework – personality, support structure, previous history, inheritance, culture, and all the other elements already discussed. Emotional upheavals take various forms and may manifest as observable and communicable emotions, as severe global distress, as states/complexes defined as post-traumatic stress disorders or in other ways. Although each person is unique, some patterns are discernible.

Grief

The emotions associated with grieving are to be expected in the course of a serious illness. There are a number of ways in which a patient may intensely experience loss, partly because the profile of loss changes as they move through the seasons of illness. Initially, it can be loss of time, finance and the capacity for gainful employment; later, loss of mobility, and eventually loss of the ability to exercise autonomy. Ideally, this last evolves into the highest exercise of autonomy, that of handing oneself over to the kindness of strangers. In such serious situations of potential or actual loss, it is important for the professional carer to ensure not only good symptom relief but also, as far as is possible, the retention of highly significant personal capacities (speech, cognition, recognition, continence) even in the last days of life.[24] Research into the latter is relatively simple and may be of more value than complex quality of life indices.

Fear

Loss and grieving do not necessarily take centre stage in the array of emotions of a seriously ill person. Fear can, though, and fear is not easy to investigate. An informal study of elderly patients in an ambulatory care clinic showed that unless they were depressed they had no difficulty in formulating things they would like to be able to do. However, when the investigators attempted to look at the obverse side of the coin and asked them to indicate what they most feared, it quickly became clear that this question caused much distress and the study was aborted within a day of commencement. The naming of fears is distressing, whereas the articulation of hopes appeared to be a pleasant task.[25]

Nevertheless, it is easy to understand the fear of an illness recurring and this is amenable to study. Lee-Jones and colleagues have reviewed this field and suggested a model in which 'stimuli, both external and internal play a role in activating cognitive responses associated with fears of recurrence'.[26] In other words, these fears are comprised of cognitions, beliefs and emotions. They note that the possible consequences of intense fears of recurrence include anxious preoccupation, limited planning for the future, and/or misinterpretation of bodily symptoms.

Fear of death has been more extensively considered,[27] if not thought about from time immemorial, but there is less formal study of other objects of fear – those which are spoken of in consulting rooms and around dinner tables. These include fear of prolonged life, maybe against one's wishes or even in disregard of advance directives; fear of loss of core capacities; fear of pain and fear of abandonment. It is harder to get reliable data on these things because of the context in which such painful questions are asked, because of the variability of the person's fear and because of the enormous diversity in the ways that fears manifest. The 'truth' may not be discoverable.

Hope

Hope has had more prominence in health research. Hockley stressed the relationship between hope and the will to live.[28] Herth and colleagues, also in the UK, have published extensively on the role of hope in nursing in various contexts, from intensive care units to the circumstances of palliative care.[29] Nekolaichuk and Bruera define hope as 'a multidimensional life force characterised by a confident yet uncertain expectation of achieving a future good which, to the hoping person, is realistically possible and personally significant'.[30] Morse and colleagues have explored the implications for nursing of the

> seven abstract and universal components of hope: a realistic initial assessment of the predicament or threat, the envisioning of alternatives and the setting of goals, a bracing for negative outcomes, a realistic assessment of personal resources and of external conditions and resources, the solicitation of mutually supportive relationships, the continuous evaluation for signs that reinforce the selected goals, and a determination to endure.[31]

It might be expected that the content of hope, as well as its manner of articulation by very ill patients would differ markedly in affluent Western contexts and non-Western and resource-poor countries. But there is a core humanity, and hope surely has some constant components. While expectations of the particular manner of fulfilment of hopes may vary, hope is centred, in the end, and at base, on matters which are not context-determined, such as enduring love of significant others, non-abandonment and a sense of one's own intrinsic worth. What is everywhere fairly evident is that the fostering of unrealistic hope – 'of course you are cured', or 'there is no chance of recurrence', or 'this new treatment is sure to control your cancer' – may lead to despair. Clinical effort needs to be expended in helping the patient to place hope in those things which will not fail, and in the end (if there is nothing else) in his/her own intrinsic dignity.

Suffering

Distress frequently accompanies illness. If it isn't recognised, or if coping and adaptive mechanisms fail, distress can evolve into suffering. The following chapter discusses suffering which, following Cassell, is understood as a sense of personal disintegration, the feeling of 'being about to go to pieces'.[32]

Cumulative adversity

Cumulative adversity is a recognised significant factor in the etiology of psychiatric illness which may apply more generally, beyond the psychiatric context.[33] The accumulation of adverse events in the course of eventually fatal illness may add up to an unbearable burden, especially where there is reduced personal and social support. Investigators have concluded that some patients with cancer manifest the features of post-traumatic stress disorder, possibly occurring at a higher rate than in the general community.[34] (This might usefully be studied in relation to measures of cumulative adversity.)

Cancer

Cancer is increasingly a chronic illness and so the considerable corpus of research into the ways patients experience chronic disease is relevant.[35] Maybe, however, that research needs to be incorporated into the conceptual framework of cancer-as-illness. There is, concentrated in the rehabilitation literature, much knowledge of the relationship between disease, disability and handicap and which could be readily applied to persons with cancer from time of diagnosis, rather than when disability, or (worse) handicap, has been established for want of intelligent preventive measures.

There is no doubt that the subjective dimensions of the cancer trajectory need far more attention. In cancer centres, just as much intellectual effort and resources should be brought to bear on the experiential dimensions of cancer as are expended on anti-cancer treatment. These dimensions include personal and family support, and relief of symptoms and planning for care throughout the experience – whether or not death is on the horizon. This resonates with the recommendations of World Health Organisation two decades ago: distribution of resources in developed/affluent countries should be such that there is equal expenditure on palliative care as there is on anti-cancer treatment; in developing countries, 90% of all cancer expenditure should be devoted to the elements of palliative care, involving especially, but not only, pain relief.[36] It is advice which has been largely disregarded the world over.

Conclusion

The human experience of illness, at any age and in any place, is an ordinary part of the human condition – it is part of the pattern of life as we know it. The philosophical basis of the duty of care is, in the end, not law, nor contract, but the call of the other, face to face. The response required of physicians involves unfailing commitment to beneficence; to the relief of suffering in so much as it arises from factors amenable to clinical measures, and to respect and guard human dignity in every circumstance, especially in those who are the most vulnerable. These responses can be grounded in, and enhanced by, an understanding of medicine as a human science.

2

On the Shape of Human Suffering

You can hold yourself back from the sufferings of the world; this is something you are free to do and is in accord with your nature, but precisely the holding back is the only suffering that you might be able to avoid. (Kafka)

The human condition is fragile. It has always been so. In their different ways, the geological record and our most ancient stories both testify to the fact that, at the beginning of our history, there were calamities which have remained imprinted on our memory. If not by catastrophe, that early awareness of fragility would have been induced by the sheer amount of labour required for survival and by the pain and risk of child-birth. But we have remained fragile – fragility is part of the essence of the human. So, too, is that longing for transcendence to which it gives rise, that hope for a condition in which fragility is absent. Ancient cave art bears mysterious witness to that awareness of transcendence in the way it depicts a symbolic, parallel, universe in which everyday existence is given another form. Could it be that such images express how humans are driven to configure, transform or transcend the world in which we live?[1] Fraught human reality demands a search for meaning.

Our earliest poetry offers glimpses into the ambiguity inherent in human fragility. Consider, for example, the pathos of Homer's portrayal of the aged King Priam, pleading with Achilles, who killed his son Hector in battle and then humiliated the body. To regain that body, Priam reveals a courage, the more impressive for its grounding in weakness:

O God-like Achilles, have fear o' the gods, pity him too,
Thy sire also remember, having more pity on me,
Who now stoop me beneath what dread mortal ever dar'd,
Raising the hand that slew his son pitiably to kiss it.[2]

It is possible that this combination of fragility and yearning informed Genesis (Bereshit), the first book of the Hebrew scriptures, redolent of other ancient texts, yet unlike them in its emphasis on our *radical ambiguity*, so giving us one of the most poignant portrayals of the human condition. Torah scholar Aviva Zornberg understands them as documents of the beginnings of desire, the obverse of which is akin to suffering – but more of that later.[3] Meanwhile, it is the dynamic between fragility and hope, between suffering and transcendence, which frames this discussion.

*

Medical practice takes place in a privileged proximity to both human distress and human suffering, these being quite distinct experiences. Eric Cassell distinguished them some decades ago in a landmark paper in which he argued that, while both are responses to some kind of harm, suffering differs from distress in that it involves a *sense of impending personal disintegration*.[4] What causes severe distress may or may not cause suffering. For Cassell, that depends on whether 'the centre' does or does not hold, for suffering is experienced when that centre, the sense of an integrated self, fails. So defined, suffering is what is commonly recognised as a feeling of 'about to go to pieces'. Animals experience distress, both when they are physically wounded and when they are emotionally wounded in bereavement. They also experience it in anticipation, as we can see when they are in line at an abattoir. We can read the language of their distress. The term 'suffering', though, is usually reserved for persons.

Suffering is complex, both in its genesis and its alleviation. Its manifestations are protean and Cassell's account raises questions which he does not himself pose. What is the source of personal coherence? What determines whether or not the centre holds? How do we understand human continuity in time? Addressing these questions will not produce definitive answers but will be an exploration into the nature of the human, likely to produce more questions but also, hopefully, deeper understanding. And it will lead to a consideration of transcendence.

Fear of suffering and the shock and awe we experience when faced with it can almost paralyse us. Can we face the Gorgon and stare down the phenomenon in order to analyse and understand it? Inevitably, it is part of human life, deserving of both respect and comfort, yet to be prevented or relieved when possible. Perhaps we can find inspiration in Bertrand Russell's attitude to life as expressed towards the end of his life: 'Three passions, simple but overwhelmingly strong, have governed my life: the longing for love, the search for knowledge, and unbearable pity for mankind.' He went on,

> Love and knowledge, so far as they were possible, led upward toward the heavens. But always pity brought me back to earth. Echoes of cries of pain reverberate in my heart: children in famine, victims tortured by oppressors, helpless old people a hated burden to their sons, and the whole world of loneliness, poverty, and pain make a mockery of what human life should be. I long to alleviate the evil, but I cannot, and I too suffer.[5]

We who are physicians must be able to bear the weight of our shared experience of suffering, at the same time as we seek to lessen its load.

*

How, then, do we approach the subject? While contemporary medical authors have recognised the need to examine suffering, there has been a regrettable tendency amongst some to objectify and measure that which is not easily quantifiable.[6] The subjective, when it is addressed, is too often treated objectively, by means of quantitative, measurable research methods. However, to understand suffering, we need to understand what is involved in the experience of 'going to pieces' and to do so we have to take into account the primacy of the subjective, for suffering is quintessentially subjective. Considered as research, such an approach goes beyond conventional methods, in that it involves reflecting seriously on the human condition in a way which deepens compassion and effects a growth in wisdom. It would be a contribution to a development of medicine as a human science, one no longer subject to the complaint that it is without 'any remotely adequate understanding of that to which we refer as a person'.[7]

Suffering is a loss of a sense of personal coherence, but what is coherence? How does the centre hold? If we consider the topic as an aspect of the human condition, the literature is vast. Here, though, some rather disparate references in unusual places will be offered, in the hope they may contain clues as to how to consider the matter anew.

We could do well to begin with Shakespeare who, according to Harold Bloom, was the first to depict the 'inner self'. Bloom attributes to Shakespeare an understanding of human development as proceeding via the way we re-conceive ourselves – a 'self over hearing', sometimes forced on us by changing circumstances and sometimes internally driven.[8] This constant re-conceptualisation takes throughout changing roles: 'All the world's a stage and in his time a man may play many parts.'[9] Clearly, coherence can be threatened in this view of a person but Shakespeare has an insight of paramount importance for carers of the suffering: 'Give sorrow words: the grief that does not speak knits up the o'er wrought heart and bids it break.'[10]

More immediately, though, we can continue the previous chapter's discussion of Erik Erikson's theory of personal development which contains, if only by implication, an account of personal continuity (the centre) and of what it is for it to hold. Erikson understood his 'psychosocial crises' to be the dynamics of personal development but they also clearly have the potential to trigger that sense of impending personal disintegration which is the essence of suffering. It can be inferred that continuity is ensured by choosing what he called the 'favourable options' for resolving crises, choices which result in a personality characterised by trust, reasonable autonomy, initiative, capacity for effort, a sense of identity and a capacity for intimate relationships. It is the unfavourable outcomes leading to confusion, isolation and stagnation which contain the potential for suffering and disintegration of an earlier continuity. Favourable outcomes sustain a sense of the wholeness of life (which Erikson calls integrity) while unfavourable outcomes lead to despair and possibly suffering.

The concept of a 'general resistance resource', developed by the Israeli sociologist Aaron Antanovsky, furthers our understanding of conditions which promote favourable outcomes.[11] A general resistance resource is a network of supportive persons, which Antanovksy demonstrated are able to influence the outcome for individuals suffering from physically related stressors. It is, of course, commonplace to recognise that connectedness is a human good. Research regarding the beneficial effect of support groups for patients with cancer is not decisive regarding cancer outcomes, but there is no doubt that, for many, life is sweeter if genuinely supported and the burden of distress shared. But Antonovsky's point is stronger – it is that there may be an *ontological* sense in which connectivity is critical for the centre to hold throughout suffering. That idea resonates with the previously mentioned views of Charles Taylor, that

> I am a self only in relation to certain interlocutors: in relation to those conversation partners who were essential to my achieving self-definition. A self exists only within 'webs of interlocution'.[12]

The concept of a general resistance resource reveals that it is culture (in the broad sense) which influences both the shape of an individual's suffering and also its social shape – that of the suffering person together with those in closest proximity, who are notably their carers, whether informal or professional. Comfort and care is basically an interpersonal activity, which is not to dismiss that given by a loved dog, or music, or nature.

There are different ideas about how the carer relates to human suffering. Rehnstadt and Eriksson, for example, write of the need for a 'meaning-creating encounter' with the caregiver, an encounter which involves progressively 'loading' the suffering, rendering it a sign of a deepening 'understanding of life' and so alleviating it somewhat.[13] Another possibility would be to consider the caregiver as a steadying vessel like a flower pot, a bulwark against fragmentation or personal disintegration, within which the person may then more freely grope towards restoration. In similar vein, the thoughtful body of research emanating from Price and colleagues at Edmonton advanced the notion that 'holding' techniques are critical in the care of persons afflicted by shock.[14] From this followed the recognition that techniques involving touch or expressions of sympathy are for later, when it may be appropriate for emotional expression to be given to the distress being endured. The presupposition here is surely that of the primacy of coherence in the midst of that impending personal disintegration Cassell called 'suffering'.

From a quite different, but no less illuminating, perspective Mary Rawlinson offers a philosophical analysis of human suffering. The central conclusion is this:

> My argument works toward the following point: the context in which these questions have typically been asked and answered by Western philosophy, or at least a tradition extending from Plato to Kant through Christian Platonism, proves inappropriate for the treatment of suffering insofar as it fails to locate suffering with respect to the purposive activity of a human subject, identifying it instead with distance or alienation from an ideal order… [It] is the hierarchy of ends distinguishing or individuating a specific subject that provides the proper context for comprehending and treating suffering.[15]

She continues in this vein:

> we open a place for suffering wherever we own some purpose as our own; purposes that may be frustrated, ends that we may fail to meet, or possibilities that may never be realised.

A topology of suffering is then advanced:

> [suffering] may visit the individual from three directions: (i) from

43

his own body, (ii) in his relations with others, or in the theatre of intersubjective life, and (iii) with respect to his powers of self-possession, self-regulation, and production vis a vis the external world, or the arena of the will. To these directions or dimensions, there must be added a fourth that comprehends the economic relationships among the other three orders, that is the effect of suffering upon the overall organization and unity of the subject's purposive activity. Suffering in (iv), the sphere of universal alteration, presents as an attack upon the fundamental coherence of the sufferer's world.

*

We have, then, some valuable frameworks within which those charged with relieving human suffering in a medical context can explore their experience but in order to take these thoughts further, we need to integrate them with an understanding of persons. Eric Cassell listed the components of a person: 'roles, relationships, actions, behaviours, as well as a body, dreams and a transcendent dimension – a life of the spirit, however expressed or known'. He stressed that persons cannot be reduced to their parts, for

> all the aspects of personhood - the lived past, the family's lived past, culture and society, roles, the instrumental dimension, associations and relationships, the body, the unconscious mind, the political being, the secret life, the perceived future, and the transcendent being-dimension – are susceptible to damage and loss.[16]

The ecological model of a person described in the introduction is rather simpler. To briefly recapitulate: the central idea is that a person is a *relational* reality, a web of relationships in a dynamic whole, these relationships being constitutive of – not adding to – personhood. From this ecological point of view, the relations which constitute a person extend both to their present life situation and to their personal past, to what they have done and what they have experienced. They refer to how the facts have been interpreted in a personal history which continues to influence the present. A person's inheritance, both biological

44

and cultural, provides the platform on which that personal history has been constructed. This set of relations has the potential to become a closed system but a way out is offered by the vector of hope (although, as has become clear in decades of clinical practice, what a patient hopes for may be difficult or painful to articulate and may also be unpredictable). On this model, all elements are in dynamic relationships with each other for the personal process is complex and each person is unique.

The question we are asking here, though, concerns what holds these notional elements together. What makes them cohere around a centre and what enables that centre to hold? What is it that general resource networks and the articulation of purposes sustain? We need, now, to take up the theme with which we began – the theme of the *radical ambiguity* of the human condition, a theme expressed in the earliest human sources. In the Hebrew scriptures, it is expressed as the idea that we are made of both the 'dust' of the earth (*nephesh*) and 'breath' (*ruah*), which is as if it were from elsewhere. But whatever its precise articulation, the idea of this ambiguity in the constitution of the human leads to an understanding in which death is the loss of whatever it is the principle of coherence, a loss which allows that which came from earth to disintegrate and return to earth.

Philosophers, of course, have written much on the subject, both for and against this conception of our radical ambiguity, but in our human experience, there is surely the thought that there is in us both something of the material universe and something other which defies entropy during our life time and sometimes called spirit or soul. Maybe the soul is best understood in our day as the principle of personal coherence, the form of the material which during life binds the whole as one.

This does not take away the problem, but it does give it a name. The shape of the inner self is yet to be illuminated. (In the following, the question of whether the form endures the dissolution of the material is not at issue.) The question here is whether spirit, the principle of personal coherence, is powerful enough to prevent personal disintegration under extreme onslaught – and, indeed, whether it can fail to assist the centre to hold even under what some might see as minor provocation. That leads to another question: what determines, or at least influences, the shape of one's core or spirit, of one's capacity not to yield to forces which threaten personal disintegration? What modifies that capacity? Although, strictly speaking, these are questions for psychologists, we others can describe what we observe and what we experience. Further reflections on the role of spirit are in chapter 6 of this book, 'After the Decade of the Dying'.

*

When Cassell insisted that one of the proper goals of medicine was the relief of suffering, he was reacting against a version of medical practice which he saw as a travesty, one where the focus on the non-personal meant that suffering as such is overlooked, where the interest is in the objectively definable disease to the exclusion of the subjective experience of illness.

The distinction is not between the art and science of medicine. Many years ago, as a newly fledged professor and a physician immersed in cancer medicine, I argued that medicine should be more, not less scientific, if it were to meet personal needs more adequately.[17] What I meant then, though perhaps the thought was not fully formulated, was just that medicine requires a developed and sound concept of a person. Clarity of the goal is critical, but because the goal is always in relation to personal preferences, it can be defined only by the patient (or their surrogate). Armed with adequate information, reasonable strategies can be discussed for achieving that goal. A patient with newly diagnosed advanced lung cancer, for example, needs to be assisted to articulate personal goals in the knowledge that their condition is regarded as almost certainly not curable, although possibly temporarily controllable. That goal may include living until a grandchild starts school, or some other personally significant event; it may be to remain at work as a carpenter, or to play piano, to golf, or to travel to visit someone. The point is that their choice will not be predictable of the basis of the disease, but the feasibility of achieving it, or the wisdom of modifying it, may well be *defined by the disease*. Clinical decision-making, commencing with the delineation of reasonable options requires a much more nuanced approach.[18]

If the patient tells their story in terms of the past as well as the present, it will be a guide to their capacity to withstand major threats to cohesion. It may also provide clues as to what might modify that capacity, for good or ill. It is significant that sometimes the very telling is the beginning of recovery, without removing what initiated it. This points to the subtlety of the dynamic of suffering and to the fact that, fundamentally, it involves personal growth.

Frequently, there will be circumstances in which it is not possible to remove the stressor and so where the task is just to assist the suffering person to endure. Particularly important here is the research discussed above on the need for holding techniques while the stressor is present, and the advisability of avoiding more potentially intrusive gestures like touch and expressions of sympathy until that stressor has gone when emotions can be given full rein. Strength may be lent (though the lender will eventually need a loan in return). This advice is all the more important precisely because it may be hard to remember. It is especially pertinent in the rush of emotion felt by those responding to natural disasters, examples of which are rather more common than one might realise.

Removal of factors threatening personal cohesion is, of course, the stuff of much medical practice, especially in the field of palliative medicine. Pain is now relievable in most instances, although cancer-related pain is still problematic. Relief of other major symptoms is also usually possible. But no level of symptom relief can obviate all suffering, for it is not intrinsically physical, but personal. What is sometimes called existential suffering may remain, because overwhelming grief in the face of loss can be such that coherence cannot be restored. In such circumstances, the only thing to be done is to attempt to strengthen the principle of coherence. Restoration of personal integrity in the face of irremediable stressors remains the human task and the means are not new. Interpersonal solidarity remains the linchpin.

The restoration of a sense of coherence will require different means in different circumstances. In general, though, it consists in re-establishing fractured relationships which may be of various kinds.

a) Intrapersonal. Re-engagement with a self thought lost might be effected in a number of ways. It could be that the removal of horrendous pain would suffice; maybe just refreshing sleep; possibly, the release from some constraint; then again, it could be that some kind of interior renewal will lead to a rebirth of hope.

b) Interpersonal. The agency of another person, stranger or familiar, can lend strength. Alternatively, there could be a reunion and reconciliation of a pre-existing, but broken, significant relationship. This can occur in person or on the telephone.

c) Place. Returning home to a place which is critical to personal identity might be what is needed to restore coherence.

d) Objects or capacities. Something else central to sense of self or self-worth – a capacity or an object – may be what is missing.

e) History. Acknowledgement of a disparaged history or cultural affinity can assist in the restoration of coherence.

f) Meaning. The discovery of meaning in the face of incomprehension or absurdity is restorative.

The art of prognosis

The art of prognosis, of foreshadowing the future, has rightly been given renewed emphasis in the last decades.[19] The goal of prognosis should also be to relieve suffering and so to enhance human flourishing. No person should die in despair. Where fatal illness is involved, the physician can assist the patient to centre hope, not on what will in the end probably fail, but on what should not fail – the commitment to care, the relief of pain, and the recognition of the intrinsic value of the patient as a unique, irreplaceable subject of existence. No person should die perceiving themselves as a therapeutic failure or disillusioned after being sustained by an unrealistic hope engendered by a physician who thought it an act of compassion. Authentic living is surely embedded not in falsehood, but in truth. No lie is justified which separates a person from his or her own truth.

The physician should never lose sight of the person as agent. Personal flourishing will be enhanced by appreciating what this person, however weak, most wants to be able to do. That may be wholly unpredictable. A physician who is walking the walk with a very ill, possibly a steadily deteriorating, patient should be gently asking several questions. Some might be about the difficulties to be faced if relief is possible, while others could touch on their present priorities. These questions are not always easy to ask, for the questioner may have their own unspoken fears and they may surface in the presence of such frailty.[20]

> Human suffering does not amount to a physical or moral pain or a difficulty. Suffering is something like crossing a desert; it is an experience in which a person will experience evil, and yet, at the same time, will be led to discover and express the deepest meaning of one's life. This is true also for the suffering of the doctor.[21]

Medical staff and suffering

The twenty-first century has seen a focus on the suffering of the sick, but there needs to be attention, too, to the suffering of medical staff.[22] Unmourned losses (sometimes called disenfranchised grief) can affect physicians and there is much at stake if they sense that their own centre is not holding. If they are not even aware of this breaking up inside, the consequences are grave. The price of unfailing equanimity as a laudable *modus vivendi* may be very high, not only for the mental health of those concerned but also for clinical decision-making. Two recent researchers into the suffering of doctors concluded, 'We are just beginning to realise that humanising medicine depends in no small part on recovering the humanity of physicians.'[23]

One could speculate that one component of the horrendous phenomenon which ensued in German medical practice nearly a century ago was that the personal development of medical personnel did not keep pace with the renowned technical excellence of the profession. Could this imbalance have contributed to what Alexander, the observer at the Nuremberg trials, described as the 'subtle shift in the basic attitude of physicians….in the attitude to the non rehabilitatable sick' and so to the capitulation of German doctors and leading academics?

> The beginnings at first were merely a subtle shift in emphasis in the basic attitude of the physicians. It started with the acceptance of the attitude, that there is such a thing as life not worthy to be lived. This attitude in its early stages concerned itself merely with severely and chronically sick. Gradually the sphere of those to be included in this category was enlarged to encompass the socially unproductive, the ideologically unwanted, the racially unwanted and finally all non-Germans. But it is important to realise the infinitely small wedged-in lever from which this entire trend of mind received its impetus was the attitude toward the non-rehabilitable sick…[24]

The Netherlands doctors, by way of contrast, demonstrated a high degree of ethical sensitivity and resisted the slide into comparable travesties.[25] It is up to sociologists, psychologists and historians together to help us understand the etiology of such subtle shifts in attitude, but simple physicians, and especially those charged with teaching and with leadership, must continue to ponder. The current explosion of technology (especially in genetics) requires a high order of interiorised ethical sensitivity in physicians and leading edge academics lest we ever forget how once, unspeakably, the medical profession abandoned beneficence and betrayed the people.

Suffering and dignity

Restoration wrought through changes discussed above is a recovery of human dignity. There is an important qualification, though, for human dignity is also present in the midst of suffering. Dignity is intrinsic – it cannot be lost even when the relationships constitutive of a person are damaged or broken. The trace of what is there suffices to make human dignity present. It is present even when not perceived by the person themselves or by those present, should they be unmindful of dignity as an order of being rather than as an attribute or mere possibility.[26] In short, what is recovered by the above means is an internal sense of human dignity.

There is an aesthetic dimension to the relationship between human dignity and human suffering as articulated by one medical researcher: 'the ongoing moral challenge in the face of pain and suffering is to ensure that our various expressions of the beautiful life continue to preserve and enhance the dignity we all share'.[27] Another writer on these topics, a professor of anatomy, wrote, 'it is the task of medicine to emancipate man's interior splendour'.[28] This may never be more true than in the face of human suffering. The nature of that splendour will remain a riddle for the mind, no matter what else we know or understand.

3

On the Kindness of Strangers:
Notes on the Experience of Care[1]

Australia, it has been suggested, is a 50,000-year-long 'ongoing conversation',[2] much of it between those who were initially strangers, but who nevertheless encountered each other as possessors of a common humanity. That sense of human connectedness is thought be a primordial response to other humans, especially to those in need.[3] While relationships between strangers are not always congenial, they are fundamental to our human infrastructure, nowhere more so than in the health system. An understanding of the concept of care which underpins that system can contribute to making those relationships harmonious.

There is a host of questions which can only be properly addressed if we have a grounding in the concept of care. What is the basis of our response to a needy other? What is the duty of care? What are the rights of the weak to receive care? Are there grounds for placing limits on care? Whether implicit or explicit, these questions are present in mainstream medical care, in end-of-life care in acute hospitals, in emergency departments and intensive care units, and above all, in community practice. They are questions which cannot be answered by empirical evidence alone. Communal reflection is called for. Advance care directives, so important to those who make them, are but one indication that patients may have a clearer view of what is their 'good' than the most senior of clinicians.

The ethics of care

The branch of ethics known as the ethics of care departs from a relational view of the human person. Care is understood to be a given in human existence, an activity that 'weaves' people into a fundamental 'network of relationships'.[4] Can the clinician contribute to this branch of the Western philosophical tradition? We have a privileged perspective in that we are very experienced in dealing with the human condition. The ecological view of a person (developed in previous chapters) is the product of that experience. On that view, a person is understood to be *constituted* by a web of relationships, a web comprised of the present environment, the past as it was experienced, and an inheritance with both biological and cultural dimensions. Whether or not the web is open or closed depends on whether the person experiences hope or despair, the latter making for a closed system, the former providing a way out of that closure.

This relational account of a person applies to carers as much as it does to patients and their support networks, for care is fundamentally an interpersonal activity, even when therapeutic interventions are largely technical:

> Care is one way of acknowledging the other as person. Care is not a corollary to rational consideration: rather it starts with respect for the other's dignity and seeing the other as person, as mystery.[5]

Such ideas, although not often expressed in words in the everyday world of clinical practice, do not preclude, but rather mandate, urgent focused attention on a wounded or failing body. In triage situations, it may be the significance of each human person within one's gaze which drives the passion to care, although the objective aspects of the human person (the vital signs and so on) are the immediate concern.

One exponent of the ethics of care defines care as follows:

> On the most general level, we suggest that caring be viewed as a species activity that includes everything that we do to maintain, continue, and repair our 'world' so that we can live in it as well as

possible. That world includes our bodies, our selves, and our environment, all of which we seek to interweave in a complex, life-sustaining web.[6]

Care of many kinds involves strangers, especially the care of our failing bodies, the immediate focus of most medical practitioners. But that care is just an instance of a larger pattern of human activity, involving so often, at its heart, the kindness of strangers. Care is an attitude and a practice, both pervasive in human communities and finely focused in the health care system. They are, indeed, the drivers of the planning, administration and evaluation of clinical activity.

Why is care needed? There are two fundamental reasons why individuals need to give and to receive care: first, we are radically incomplete, and second, we experience trauma and/or loss as normal components of human life. We could add a third: 'interdependency as an ineliminable feature of human social existence'.[7]

Our radical incompleteness stems not merely from biological need but from the fact that, as persons, we are constituted by our relations. Baby birds need mothers or fathers to care for them or they will die. Humans need far more than food, water and shelter. To grow as persons we need others: 'of these one and all I weave the song of myself'.[8] We not only exist, but also grow, in what Taylor called 'webs of interlocution', a process which necessarily involves the experience of illness and loss.[9]

Some French revolutionaries entertained the possibility of the elimination of death.[10] Sometimes, at Grand Rounds, zealous junior medical staff would seem to almost share that goal. But death is universal, part of the human pattern, and just as the last movement of a symphony contributes richly to the shape of the whole, so is death part of the shaping of human life. Trauma/loss/distress and/or frailty are normal parts of the human condition, however much we seek to prevent and alleviate them.

Why care for another? Care of some kind is manifest in all human communities. Is the capacity innate in human beings? Indeed, is it innate more widely? In observing a colony of non-human primates, one can see manifestations of caring behaviour; moreover, in many species, the bonding of mothers for their newborn babies appears to be instinctive. There is more than this, though, with humans. Desmond Manderson, drawing on the philosophy of Emanuel Levinas, grounds the duty of care in 'the call of the other'.[11] Only this call of the other is strong enough to sustain a physician or nurse responding day after day to situations of distress. Nothing else could drive those involved in caring for people in unspeakable situations such as wars and civil disasters.

However, the recognition of the power of the call of the other in need raises the question of the limits to care and of the need to set boundaries (especially for junior clinical staff) and also of the delineation of the principles upon which these boundaries may be ethically drawn. Boundaries are necessary because the caring self is an other to oneself, an other also in need of care.[12] Care of the self is mandated for oneself in order that one may care for the other. The self lives to respond to the other, and for this reason, care requires attention to the self. This is not narcissism but radical altruism and its implications need careful teasing out in the context of health care. The stress experienced by carers of all types of very ill patients may be extreme, and both clarity of thought and principles of practice are needed. Clinical decision-making should always include consideration of carer impact, though often it does not.

Clinical decision-making in complex situations: some implications of the foregoing with special reference to palliative medicine[13]

As an area of clinical science and practice, palliative medicine has several components:

a) symptom relief in parallel with anti-disease strategies, both now resting on a sound basis of clinical science

b) providing assistance to, or enabling, personal and family support as needed

c) participation in clinical decision-making, preferably from the time of the diagnosis of the probably fatal illness.

Palliative care, as distinct from palliative medicine, involves planning for future care and approaching death, aftercare for bereaved persons, and a number of other matters. A useful discussion was published in 1997 by the Institute of Medicine based in Washington DC as a response to travesties in end-of-life care, brought to light in (then) recent clinical research. The report recommended that palliative care should begin with the diagnosis of the eventually fatal illness and then be subject to what it called 'mixed management', meaning that all aspects of palliative care should be available to all diagnosed patients, whether or not specialist palliative care professionals were involved.[14] The implications of mixed management are not confined to palliative care but clearly also relate to the practice of palliative medicine, including its education and training and research.[15] If the mixed management – we could simply say integrated – approach prevails, the evaluation of end-of-life care, at least in terms of outcome measures, should not usually distinguish between the different contributions of palliative care services. This is a significant shift. The involvement in clinical decision-making of persons with clear perspectives but not necessarily specialised competence in palliative care is a welcome and wise development.[16]

Specialist palliative care resources (its textbooks, journals and websites) are full of information about how to assess patients, techniques for pain and symptom relief, approaches to the care of patients in special circumstances, ideas for organising care, and so on. However, the subject of clinical decision-making warrants more attention. Decisions punctuate the experience of illness for both patient and physician. Almost every hour of every day, decisions are made by those charged with the care of seriously ill patients. There are countless matters to decide: which investigation to conduct; which treatment approach to adopt; which consultation procedures are appropriate; what manner of communication is best. Some decisions are easy, being almost automatic and according to established protocol, while others require various levels of scrutiny.

Whether these decisions are right or wrong, they can have a profound impact on both the patient and their carers. They also impact on the administrators of finite resources.

When a patient is in the last phase of life, clinical decision-making can be particularly fraught – the more so, if the patient is approaching death. Along with the technical aspects of palliative medicine, matters to be decided in such circumstances may involve difficult and complex ethical questions, such as how to balance competing strategies and when, and how, to allow a patient to die rather than persisting in prolonging their life.

Clearly there is need for a methodology which can be applied almost instinctively in such demanding and complex situations – one, which ideally, would be internalised in the course of medical education. How can this be approached? Certainly, philosophical ethics as such could be given more attention in medical schools.[17] But it is not ethicists who make the decisions in everyday clinical practice and heightened ethical competence may be required of physicians now. The ecological view of a person grounds a relatively simple approach which embodies the central ethical traditions without labelling them as such.

Clinical decision-making requires first, clarification of the reasonable options under the prevailing circumstances. At this point, input is needed about the objective aspects of the patient's condition, and also about the individual and subjective dimensions of their situation. Relevant legal requirements and resource restraints must also be determined. It cannot be wise, and nor is it mandatory, to place on the table all possible (even experimental) options. Respect for the patient's autonomy does not demand that. So judgement should be exercised in the initial choice of options advanced for consideration.

Thereafter, each reasonable option may be considered systematically in terms of traditional ethical principles.

a) The principle of autonomy requires determining the preferences of the (appropriately informed) patient and their family.

b) The principle of beneficence demands consideration of the benefits to be expected from a course of action and the likelihood of these being achieved.

c) The principle of non-maleficence requires assessing the risk of the harm.

d) The principle of justice involves asking whether the proposed course of action is fair to the patient and to the others concerned (carers/family/hospital/community).

Controversy surrounds the interpretation of these principles which, narrowly interpreted, are not adequate bases for decision-making. Progress can be made, however, if we elaborate them in terms of an adequate view of personhood. The resulting understanding not only advances a relational interpretation of these principles, but also incorporates an understanding of the relation between them. For example, in recognising the human capacity to make wise judgement in situations of complexity, there is an acknowledgement of the notion of virtue as understood in virtue ethics. There is an element of deontological ethics in the recognition of the influence of prevailing values, and an aspect of consequentialism in the imperative to carefully examine not only the merits of the strategies under consideration but also their foreshadowed outcomes.

Such an elaboration is especially helpful in applying the principle of autonomy and its concretisation in the requirement of informed consent. If a person is a relational reality, consent needs to be far more than an individual saying yes to a proposal. The following considerations need to be addressed. What information is essential for the consent to be valid? What information is necessary to ensure that consent is not under duress? If, as T.S Eliot wrote, 'Man cannot bear too much reality', how much reality is necessary for the patient for their consent be authentically in accord with their values, lived life, history, culture, current environment/relationships? Should the patient understand the implications for others of the giving or withholding of consent?

Some of the underlying philosophical ideas here have recently been articulated by Jeff Malpas:

> It is not that autonomy has no relevance to an understanding of human being, but rather that too great an emphasis on autonomy alone threatens to deliver a distorted picture of that in which a human being consists. Who and what we are is not determined solely by our existence as independent beings, but is instead intertwined with the being of those others to whom our lives are shaped, as well as with respect to the wider world in which our lives are played out... If the principles that determine human being are indeed principles of relationality that place human thinking and acting in an ever-present relation of interdependence with others and with the world, then to think and act autonomously will not be to think and act in separation from others and the world, but to think and act in a way that is attentive to them.[18]

Discussion about strategy is vitiated by unclear goals. Goal setting requires care. Generic concepts such as relief of suffering or prolongation of life need to be more precisely defined for an individual patient who is in a particular time and place and state. Attention should be given to the values prevailing in those particular circumstances and cultural climate, these forming, as it were, a moral horizon. They include such things as the value of life; human dignity; human possibility; the value of last phase of life and of dying; privacy; human fraternity, liberty, and equality; and other matters held dear.

Care needs to be taken to avoid flat-of-the-curve medicine which results in diminishing benefit and increasing expenditure of resources which include time and energy.[19] Physicians, especially, need to be alert to those options which are clearly at the flat part of the curve. There are some aspects of cancer care which can bring high yield in return for resources used – pain relief, for example, closely followed by surgery, radiotherapy or chemotherapy. On the other hand, there are some circumstances where the ratio of benefit to resources is not so high and some where the more that is done, the greater the distress of the patients. Nevertheless, working at the flat of the curve is justifiable in carefully monitored research settings because they may throw light on how advances can be made.

There is another point worth noting. In criminal cases, verdicts are delivered on the basis of 'beyond reasonable doubt', while in civil cases the ground is 'on the balance of probabilities'. It is the latter standard which pertains to clinical decisions which leaves open the possibility of error, despite all care. We must be prepared to cope with making errors.

Clinical decision-making occurs on the basis of medical and legal considerations, resource limitations and social facts. Although they have received comparatively little attention, social facts are significant, as they are relevant to the social consequences of a course of action. As already mentioned, there is a case for carer impact statements, something like the environmental impact statements which are prepared in relation to major building constructions. Carer impact statements would outline the likely effect of a treatment on carers and/or families and so could well affect decisions about, say, prolonging life or moving patients from one facility to another.

For example, an attempt to prolong life for a week or two by another course of chemotherapy, with a five to ten per cent chance of the disease responding and an eighty per cent chance of severe side-effects may seem to be an acceptable proposal at first sight but might appear less so when the burden on those whom the patient loves is taken into account. It could be that the patient has considered others all their life and would very much want to do so now, at this fraught time. Is it ethical to withhold impact-others information?

It needs to be kept in mind when striving for evidence-based medicine, that not all that is known has been written down in Western European languages, and not all that has been written in these languages has been considered by those formulating statements regarding evidence. Since, further, the individual aspects of patients are deliberately suppressed in clinical trials, the continuing narrowing down of evidence needs to be kept in mind. There is no evidence as to the benefit or harm likely to ensue from a proposed course of action, for evidence relates to the efficacy of clinical manoeuvres and is part of the fact base for the decision, not the decision itself. Evidence is not, in itself, judgement or wisdom.

In the face of all of these elements of a complex ecological situation, a decision usually has to be made about the wisest choice of available options. This exercise of judgement requires professional integrity, manifest as clinical wisdom. A judgement that a specified course of action would be futile is a judgement the patient may need to make in the light of appropriate information. On the other hand, a physician cannot be obliged to implement a decision which he or she considers, on balance, to be unwise, or simply wrong. Patient autonomy is not the only autonomy at stake.

Certainly, the way we choose to live the last weeks or days of life is as diverse as the way we choose to live other periods of life. There is no correct way to die. (The teaching of *ars moriendi* in past times did not fully recognise that.) King Lear rejected attempts to avert his death:

> O let him pass, he hates him,
> That would upon the rack of this tough world
> Stretch him out longer

On the other hand, Dylan Thomas urges us to 'Rage, rage, against the dying of the light.'

The dignity of difference in this and all things is to be celebrated. It is not the role or responsibility of professional carers to attempt to change such preferences, though it may be their responsibility to ensure that the patient has access to the appropriate understanding of that impact and the impact of alternative treatment options. They are responsible, too, to see that there is adequate consideration given to the impact of the treatment options on others. Those kinds of information can be hard to impart gently but should not be withheld.

Obviously, complex matters have been oversimplified here. Nevertheless, a conscientious, even if brief, systematic consideration of the sensible options may offer a way through a difficult morass, and assist patients and professionals under stress. At the very least, the reasons for a very difficult decision will have been articulated, perhaps in writing, available, then, for later consideration if the outcome appears to have been either unsatisfactory or unanticipated. As Karl Popper stressed, the careful examination of error is a tool for the advancement of knowledge.[20]

An overarching ethical principle should be imprinted in the mind of physicians charged with the care of those with an eventually incurable illness. Over the years, I have been guided by the traditional Jewish ethic: Affirm life! But do not obstruct death! Furthermore, a just society embodies a fundamental ethic, namely that care of the weak is mandatory; they are to be valued and cared for.[21] It may be timely to note again the analysis of Leo Alexander at the Nuremberg trials, that the travesties of the medical profession arose from an initial devaluing of the incurably ill, the weakest in society, with that 'subtle shift in emphasis, the acceptance of the attitude, that there is such a thing as life not worthy to be lived. This attitude in its early stages concerned itself merely with severely and chronically sick.'[22]

'The longest journey is the journey inward' and we may come to see that the rock to which we journey is within ourselves, our human core, and that one day we will know it, and enter into it, and stay there.[23] If this is the fundamental personal reality, our care systems have much to safeguard and to cherish.

In conclusion

At the heart of Australia is a rock – Uluru. The seeking of the centre is a constant in Australian culture.[24] The most difficult journey for the discipline of medicine in Australia may be the exploration of its own core. It may be that there are Australian nuances to the concept of person which are yet to be appreciated arising, perhaps, from the chequered long history of humankind in this place; the kaleidoscope of cultural patterns; the hidden personal and collective often hidden grieving; and the relationship to the painful beauty of the land. Maybe, too, the kindness of strangers, the giving and receiving of it, is part of our inheritance and a principle of our hope.

Part Two

4

Diagnosis and Prognosis

Background

A medical intervention is a drama. It may be straightforward and felicitous or it may be harrowing. There are several actors involved -- the patient, his/her seconds, the doctor and his/her team, maybe onlookers of various categories (such as prompters and interpreters) and administrators/funders. All of these need to be taken into account if the action is to be understood and the drama evaluated. As is the case in theatre, movies or operas, the wider cultural context has a bearing on how the drama is interpreted.

There are many ways of understanding the relationship between patients and health professionals (especially physicians). They emerge in response to circumstances and cultural tides and so are subject to fashion. Since the health care policies of many developed countries are now formulated in circumstances which are quite fraught, the principles and values involved warrant thorough examination. Over and above the debates about health care insurance and the role of funders in shaping clinical decisions, there is the issue of the level of individual care and this requires urgent scrutiny.

When physicians become patients, they share their experience and their fears. Some experienced doctors who have been laid low by serious illness have been articulate in their criticisms of the competence of their carers (including physicians) as decision-makers and comforters.[1] Many have been found to be neither humble nor wise. Do such painful-to-read contributions receive the attention they merit? Where do such anecdotes of core deficiencies fit in the spectrum of medical evidence? Karl Popper, who recognised error as a powerful tool for the advancement of learning, may well have regarded such testimonies as more important than the countless expressions of gratitude confirming the hypothesis that, on the whole, care is satisfactory. Outcome evaluation based on search for error may yield more than measures of praise, even in a busy hospital practice.

There is further reason for disquiet. As far back as 1978, Alain Enthoven was arguing the need to avoid flat-of-the-curve medicine where the yield in benefit is not proportionate to the huge costs involved.[2] For the patient, who is the ultimate judge of benefit and cost, flat-of-the-curve medicine can be disastrous because opportunities to increase suffering rather than alleviate it are multiplied. The individual physician, who may be enthusiasm-rich and time-poor, needs to take care that actions with high benefit-to-cost ratio (such as pain relief for patients with cancer) are not neglected in favour of measures at the flat of the curve. There is a place for research into investigative therapies with a low chance of useful response but there should also be a clear understanding that priority in resources needs to be assured for the high-benefit aspects of practice. There is also room for more research to establish more adequate measures of benefit and cost. As well, there should be constant efforts in clinical practice to reduce the cost (for example by less toxic and tailored therapies) and to maximise the benefit by such things as good care, symptom relief throughout treatment, and rehabilitation. Strategies to reduce the price of benefit should involve all physicians in contact with patients who have a probably fatal illness.

The art of diagnosis

The role of physicians, compared with those of their other professional colleagues, can be seen to be primarily analytic, even diagnostic. Their job is to first define the problem for this person in the here and now and then to recommend what intervention, if any, should be undertaken and by whom. Following that, they need to suggest preventive measures in an order of priority and finally they need to evaluate the success or failure of interventions.

This analytic/diagnostic activity should be based on some fundamental principles. The first of these is that a person is a relational being, as briefly elaborated below (and extensively in earlier chapters); the second is that beneficence is the overriding aim, with the recognition that what is the good for a patient is normally perceived by them better than by others; the third is that other persons may be needed to improve the quality of the diagnosis/appraisal with respect to one or more of its aspects. All of these principles may need to be qualified. For example, beneficence may occasionally be consistent with – or require – a benign paternalism. This should be recognised as such by the paternalist, who is usually the doctor. This is because it is in need of informal, if not formal, justification and may or may not bear the scrutiny of the patient, the community or professional peers.

All enlightened clinicians recognise that a patient cannot be adequately considered as a case of X disease, for the disease does not exist except in relation to this person's body or mind, other than an abstract intellectual construct. The fact that a person is a relational reality means more than this. It means that he or she is constituted by relationships with other persons, from the past and in the present, and that she or he is embedded in a cultural matrix and is encountered as such. This is the truth and richness of the human condition, the stuff of suffering as well as joy, of fear as well as meaning and hope. This has to be perceived, at least inchoately, even if not clearly articulated. Ideas like these are the substrate on which clinical understanding and adequate diagnoses can be built: the physician as diagnostician is logically a forerunner to any notion of the physician as healer.

Diagnostic activity should involve due recognition of the patient's own priorities. These may be focused on the relief of a particular symptom, on an appropriate investigation, or on the need for a certain aspect of care. It is both more respectful and more efficient for the patient to volunteer their perceived needs than it is for a physician (or any associated colleagues) to intrude into unnamed territories. This is especially significant in the face of complex issues like demoralisation, distress, suffering or spirituality. It may be that the only assistance the patient requests is some help with pain relief and that any attempt to introduce other matters into a consultation by a primary or specialist physician would be inappropriately invasive and presumptuous. On the other hand, there is data to suggest that some patients appreciate the assistance of a competent physician in such matters.

Clearly, each physician needs to reflect deeply on these questions and to be prepared to modify their role according to circumstance. Further, they need to recognise the limits of their own competence. While it is rarely appropriate for a physician to volunteer a poor prognosis to a patient, there is a responsibility to create a space for the patient to ask appropriate questions and to receive truthful answers. Lack of sensitivity to how the physician's role can be matched to the patient's needs can seriously compromise the benefit of their intervention, if not increase the distress of a vulnerable patient (and/or their family).

Analysis needs to go deep – it needs to unravel the etiology of distress, to identify the available options for altering the course of the disease and to think about how symptoms may be improved, whether or not the disease can be controlled. A solid understanding of the pathogenesis and pathophysiology of the disease should also assist in assessing problems likely to arise. The clinician should ask what is on the horizon? Are acute complications to be expected? What can be anticipated to reduce consequent distress?

Are there cultural implications of the present situation which need particular attention in the present and are there likely to be such in the future? There is more to culture than ethnicity, for it includes historical facts like trauma from war or imprisonment; the current geographic situation; economic hardship; and occupational factors. The cultural gap between doctor and patient may be very great, not only in social and economic status but also in lifetime experience and in world view, namely in the understanding of life, illness, death, suffering and the cosmos. There may be a different weighting placed on relevant personal tasks. The interpersonal gap between a sincere and competent young physician, intent on achieving excellence and maybe establishing a family, and an elderly person facing fragility or death may be unbridgeable by any training. It is a yawning gap which cries out for recognition and a sense of a common humanity.

There are different ideals of the doctor/patient relationship. It can be seen as a partnership or, as in past times, the doctor can be understood as the servant of the ill. Then again, there is the notion that the patient is a guest in the doctor's sphere of activity – a guest to be received with the kindness and respect associated with traditional hospitality. But maybe it is the physician who is a guest in the patient's presence, having been invited into a place where he or she is alien but welcome. If so, the doctor must recognise the responsibilities of a guest and respect the boundaries of that mystery which the patient always truly remains. What difference would it make to a clinical or hospital ward if it is the doctor and not the patient who is the guest, the patient then being the host? That arrangement would not be a glorification of power or autonomy, but rather the recognition of the diversity of the human condition which is just another facet of human interdependence.

Diagnostic activity involves assessing the need to involve professionals with complementary skills to one's own. Consider, for example, a case with severe symptoms which prove difficult to relieve without cumbersome drug side-effects. What if there is a lack of clinical information, even prognostic information? Or if the patient experiences untoward global distress? Or a family dysfunction interferes with care? Maybe there are complicated ethical issues. Various types of specialists are relevant to these cases and it is the responsibility of a physician, especially a primary physician, to specify the problem as precisely as possible in order to obtain the correct referral. The competence of colleagues in nursing, physiotherapy, social work and other cognate professions ordinarily far exceeds medical competence in some specific areas. The physician needs only to be assured of agreed sensible goals and how those goals will be evaluated, leaving the strategies to be applied to the relevant non-medical colleagues.

The clinician has to judge whether referral to a palliative medicine specialist is appropriate. If needed, but not readily available (which may be an acute hospital, a nursing home or a private home), the task is to recommend the next best alternative. This could be to organise telephone assistance, arrange attendance at a palliative medicine clinic, or to seek admission to a special facility. It should be expected of of all physicians that they have the competence first, to recognise poor symptom relief, and second, not to accept poor pain relief either as inevitable or as something which can be treated by anti-disease strategies alone. Anti-cancer therapy is not usually the primary solution to pain in cancer. For cancer pain, analgesic treatment is mandatory, whether or not anti-disease strategies are available and appropriate. (The error unfortunately still prevails in some contexts.) It is to be stressed that palliative care is able to be given by a variety of persons and is not to be equated with specialist palliative care services. (These are not available in many countries and may be patchy even where widespread availability of consultative services is the national goal.)

The aphorisms of the Hippocratic tradition include this: 'The physician must not only be prepared to do what is right himself, but also to make the patient, the attendants and externals cooperate.' In other words, Hippocrates saw the physician as the regulator or controller of the whole enterprise. That view may not fit the ethos of interdisciplinary teams but it may be helpful for discussions to refer to the schema in The Care Pyramid opposite. This is an inverted pyramid which recognises the critical role of the physician, whether s/he is the primary physician, the specialist in disciplines related to the disease in question, or the specialist in palliative medicine. (The role may be critical but it is a minor one overall.)

It has already been noted that the physician who is based in the community has particular advantages with respect to several dimensions

The Care Pyramid
(For patients with eventually fatal illness,
especially when approaching death)

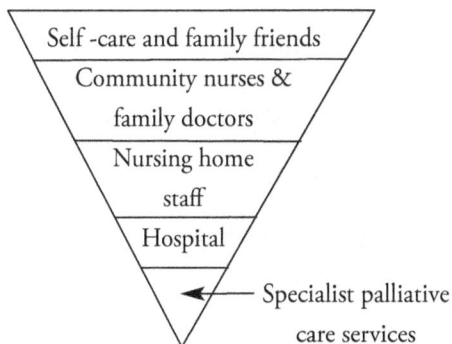

Self -care and family friends
Community nurses &
family doctors
Nursing home
staff
Hospital

Specialist palliative
care services

of medical practice. The breadth of opportunities, and the comprehensiveness of the knowledge of the community-based practitioner may need to be supplemented at times by the less comprehensive but more focused competence of a hospital-based palliative medicine specialist.

It is to be noted that specialist palliative medicine and other persons in a specialist palliative care team are at the base, not the apex, of the care pyramid. This is because their role should be seen as supportive of the whole enterprise, available when the more visible and usual means of care prove insufficient or inadequate. For the latter have no claim to moral high ground or excellence in communication though they are charged with having higher levels of critically needed competence in the understanding and relief of major symptoms, or of existential distress, or the resolving of complex ethical situations.

The specialist in palliative medicine is, then, a tiny part of the spectrum of activity of involved physicians. They should be always supportive and at times they are needed specifically. In such a framework, the contribution of the palliative medicine specialist should not be separated out from the whole enterprise – for example, for research purposes. Rather, their contribution may be best seen as a means of merging efforts and assisting in the cohesiveness of care. This is, of course, only in situations of affluence, not when doctors are a rare and scarce commodity.

This way of considering the complexity of care accords well with the mixed management called for by a landmark report of the Institute of Medicine. (The term parallel care is more favoured in Australia.) The ramifications are far reaching for a physician's self-understanding, for medical education, clinical practice, administration and funding as well as for research.

Approaching clinical decision-making

Diagnosis, in the broadest sense, underpins options about what is best to do. Clinical decisions usually involve a choice of options in the face of several alternatives. There is a vast literature on medical ethics and on the more narrowly focused clinical ethics, but even so, there may be value in outlining an approach which might help physicians charged with navigating in a sea of difficulties and often in emotionally charged circumstances.

Clinicians are faced with significant, and often difficult, decisions virtually every hour of the working day, frequently late at night and in emergency situations. It is essential that the processes of decision-making are facilitated and underpinned by the internalisation of key relevant philosophical, legal and ethical principles so that a balanced approach becomes intuitive. Sound clinical decision-making and practice may then contribute to human flourishing and community cohesiveness. An ecological framework for decision-making may be of practical assistance. Physicians are not alone, for they are in the presence of the legacies of human thought and experience, the more relevant because they are embedded in a rich stream of human activity. In the context of the care of those approaching death, the traditional Jewish ethic of affirming life but not obstructing death may be a guide to wise decisions.

The ecological approach to clinical decision-making was developed in the course of practice and teaching in Sydney teaching hospitals. It was based on

a) a concept of cost/benefit analysis, with recognition of the complexity of the costs and benefits under scrutiny

b) an adequate philosophical anthropology – the ecological view of the person which takes into account current environment, personal history, inheritance (biological and cultural)

c) an amalgam of features of some ethical traditions. It emphasises the complexity of the personal.

It takes note of the values in the air (conditioned by historical and cultural factors, and worthy subjects of research), of the factual basis (medical, including evidence base, relevant law, and resource limitations) and analysis of the implications of autonomy, beneficence, non-maleficence and justice (individual and social). The central task remains that of making a decision, on the balance of probabilities, by exercising wisdom. Such an ecological portrayal of the process of decision-making emphasises the complexity of the personal.

This approach appears to be have been welcomed by medical students as well as by graduates as a useful piece of furniture for the mind, and also as a basis for discussion, research and further refinement. Attention to the various aspects of this model need to become intuitive if such an approach is to be a practical clinical tool.

We cannot be sure of all of the facts, or judgements, or perspectives, or consistent wishes of any fellow person in his or her whole-life context, but we can be sure whether or not every reasonable effort has been made to reach the best understanding. In everyday clinical practice, many far-reaching decisions must be made quickly. The classic situation is in the emergency room, but rapid decisions are needed in hospital wards, nursing homes and private homes. And so it is with driving cars in heavy traffic. The only sound approach is the considered, deliberate internalisation of an ethical instinct (traffic sense), by painstaking education and reflection in clinical contexts. Then, the rapid responses in situations of extreme urgency and complexity will be wise and usually correct in the circumstances.

In this model, issues such as decisions on behalf of incompetent patients, are seen as part of life narratives, not as arguments to be won by set procedures, or victories for principles (or worse, for persons other than the patient). The fact of uncertainty has to be part of the whole dynamic.

The exercise of wisdom by physicians implies perceiving lines in the sand beyond which we should not go. The ethical instincts of beneficent, experienced, good persons (including clinicians) can do this. Consideration should be given to the implications of moving the line in the sand. For example, the question of reproducing humans, not as an end but as a means to another's good as in the fourth transplant of Kazuo Ishiguro's novel *Never Let Me Go*, is a radical departure from a Kantian ethic in that individuals are prepared from birth to be total organ donors. Is this a line in the sand not to be crossed? Such situations are not encountered in this form in the context of the care of seriously ill patients at present, but could well appear in the future – items, then, on the list of technically possible options for life prolongation. It has already been pointed out that major aberrations can flow from the almost unnoticeable (at the time) pushing of the envelope, from what Alexander called a 'shift in attitude to the non-rehabilitatable sick'. Furthermore, 'social justice as well as individual justice has been listed as one of the principles to be considered in clinical decision-making'.

Prognosis

Prognosis, the foretelling of what is likely to happen to this person, with this illness, in this context, is a core medical task. (Once, it was the predominant, if not almost the only, medical task, as is evident in the writings of Hippocrates.) Recently there has been a burgeoning of monographs, journal articles, reviews and research on the subject.[3] The transmission of prognosis to the patient is for the sake of assisting them in shaping their activity and possibly their priorities. While a careful prognosis may assist carers and also health services, this is a secondary, though still significant, benefit.

Making the best estimate of length of life is a serious matter. The force of mortality is such that we will all die. Acceptance this fact both for oneself and for one's patients is a considerable challenge.

However, there is far more than likely survival time involved in determining what is likely to happen. Survival time is one dimension of prognosis and for many patients: it may be far from the most important (even if some reports of clinical trials give the contrary impression). The question is what the future is likely to hold for this individual patient with an eventually fatal illness. Here, the term quality of life is very limited in its usefulness. What needs to be estimated is expected pattern of symptoms; the probability of their reasonable control and by what means; their expected interference with function, especially those functions which are critical for this individual patient; a profile of future care needs and how best they can be met; and so on. And there is the crucial prediction, sometimes in response to a precise question: 'How will I die doctor?' 'What will be happening at the end?'

The communication of prognosis must first of all be based on a sound grasp of the medical and personal facts. This requires an understanding of

a) the pathophysiology of the disease and the realistic possibility of response to further treatment

b) the history of the evolution of the disease, and its response to treatment, to this point

c) the personal response of this patient to the illness thus far, and current priorities for action and reasonable targets for achievement

d) the current agreed clinical plan, based on sound decision-making

e) the resources available for care.

With due regard for the facts of the situation, there is a chance for sensitive communication which will support this patient in what may be a painful struggle to face the future. Without that, it is possible to add to the patient's distress. Experience (level 4 evidence!) suggests that a boundary concept may be useful. This involves (especially when discussing likely survival time) the following:

• first of all, stressing the fact of uncertainty. Doctors do not know everything and predictions may not be correct. Nevertheless, they must try.

• naming a future time before which you do not really expect any drama: 'I/we would be surprised if you actually died in the next week/month/ three months/year.'

• naming an outer boundary beyond which you would be very surprised if the patient survived: 'On the other hand I/we might be surprised if we are still discussing this in, say a week, a month, three months, a year, three years, five years.'

• supporting this patient with strong eye contact when you name that outer boundary, because it may be very painful for them hearing it stated.

• supporting, also, those closest to that patient, either if they are present during this communication or if you see them afterwards.

Above all, remember that prognosis is a privileged inter-personal communication. It is a communication from one person with high levels of information, knowledge, competence, and maybe power, to another in a very different situation. Even if the recipient is another doctor, the difference is extreme.

Human complexity is to be respected always, both in oneself and in another. If this is not remembered, and in humility, we can make mistakes. Be careful! Sometimes poetry has something to offer.

To a Conscientious Prognosticator

You know, you say, what will happen –
you know the way ahead of me, can tell
the shape of shadows, lineaments of darkness,
storm and stress, the form of the trajectory,
and even according to a validated
formula published in a high impact
journal space, my time tracks, and count
my chance of life, the odds of being here,
or there, or wherever – if I care to know.
What do you know? Only what you
can measure on your paltry scales –
not what sustains my heart, kindles
the embers of my mind's fires,
livens my dust, slakes my thirst,
furnishes my dreams and holds me
till the fountain yields within me.

You know the frame, the boundaries
of the flawed art of my life piece,
that's all – and the soft score marks
of a symphony incomplete, my song still
still unsung.
Oh look, can you yet listen!

Part Three

5

Living in the Decade of the Dying

Recently, at Grand Rounds at a teaching hospital, I learned that the age at which most people in Australia die is in the decade seventy-five to eighty-five years. Since I am living in that decade, this information prompted renewed reflection. There is much written about morbidity in the aged, the causes and processes of their dying and their need for end-of-life care. But what of the experience of living in this decade? It is rather like being a marathon runner who has heard the bell, is knowingly facing the last lap and welcoming gentle cheering from the onlookers, but finishing the task alone. What is it like to live in this context? The attempt here is to lay bare the perspective of a medical clinician living in the decade of the dying, hoping it may assist in the kind of personal interaction which is the mark of a true clinician.

What are the losses and gains of persons in this decade?

The losses

These occur in relation to almost all of the constitutive relations of a person as outlined in the ecological conception of a person (chapters 1, 2 and 3).

At least two of these are both obvious and almost universal – the loss of a social/occupational role and some loss of physical capacity, including energy. With respect to the second, the current enthusiasm for teams in patient care needs to be accompanied by a recognition of the effort required to relate to a new person. The involvement of numerous persons, however kindly, has the potential for wasting the patient's sparse store of energy. The presence of more than two persons at a bed-side of a critically ill patient may add to distress.

Adverse life events are frequent for persons in the decade for dying, who often become separated from significant others by death, dementia or displacement. Separation from one's culture, whether ethnic culture, occupational culture or religious culture, can be the cause of a deep grief which is not often articulated or recognised. Likewise, separation from one's past because of perceived cognitive decline creates much distress whether that decline is from natural causes or a result of drugs prescribed by conscientious but thoughtless doctors. (The current laudable concern about gross polypharmacy in the elderly needs to focus on the personal consequences and be urgently remedied.) That all of these losses can contribute to bereavement is well known. They are a normal part of human life and should not to be pathologised.

Suffering

Losses for an elderly person are often accumulative, but even singly they may lead to palpable distress and also to profound suffering in Cassell's sense of a feeling of 'impending personal disintegration' (chapter 2). Suffering, so understood, is wholly subjective and may remain hidden. Even so, it can be discerned in words or action. Clinical staff need to appreciate that suffering is a complex phenomenon which requires urgent and skilful attention. It should certainly not be labelled as the patient being difficult or as their inability to cope. It may be that the final straw which led to a sense of being about to go to pieces can be identified by sensitive questioning within a trusted relationship. Often its effect can be rectified. Maslow's account of the hierarchy of human needs in which physiological needs are the first to warrant attention is valid, but other needs, such as those for emotional security and an outlet for creative action, are also important. There is no place for trite slogans such as care of the 'whole person' (or 'holistic care') if what we mean by 'person' is not understood.

The gains

Are there any gains in the later phases of life? Yes, surely. The first is obvious – the freedom to allocate time and energy for desired pursuits, not necessarily only the legendary golf or fishing. Secondly, in the aged, cynicism is often trumped by a deep optimism. The elderly usually retain trust – trust in persons, in place and in being and this trust, such a rare commodity in our times, is less often betrayed by sheer thoughtlessness. The basic stance of the older person may mean that the news of the day, however sensational (including news about one's medical state/prognosis) is perceived against a larger backdrop, issuing in an equanimity which may surprise, even confuse, the young, including the young doctor. Further, aged persons are often capable of a growing transparency towards the close of life. Their defences have fallen away and the onlooker is rightly in awe of a certain grandeur revealed.

Awareness of oneself and of one's world is enhanced as life progresses – it is an emergent phenomenon. As an infant, one's circle of awareness is very tiny, expanding explosively in the processes of education. By adolescence, one is aware of, even tortured by, the great questions about the self, the universe, and 'all that is'. (One reviews one's adolescent poetry at one's peril.) As one moves through life, the questions become sharper and the answers may be less clear, though somehow richer, and one learns to tolerate ignorance while still searching as an explorer. There may also be a new openness, in place of that opaqueness which is often cultivated as a shield against criticism and the slings and arrows of fortune. The perspective of the elderly may have a richness that could complement the fresh ardour of the newly aware young questioner, for most older persons are both aware and content that the young are the future.

Personal tasks of those in the later decades

Previous chapters have discussed Erikson's portrayal of human life as a sequence of stages characterised by tasks, with choices made notably at times of crisis. The choices may be of favourable options – in infancy, that would mean opting for trust over distrust; in childhood, for industry over indolence; in adolescence, for intimacy over isolation; and in mid-life, for generativity rather than stagnation. And so on. The task of old age on this view is the choice between what Erikson called 'integrity' – a sense of the wholeness of life over despair and a dominant sense of regret.

There is a connection between what Erikson depicts as despair and Cassell's conception of suffering as a sense of impending personal disintegration. It is clear that the clinical context of the elderly, especially of those in hospital, is fraught with possibilities for inducing despair and suffering. It is important to understand not only the losses which may be aggravated by hospitalisation, but also the despair which may be induced in persons already rendered vulnerable by multiple loss.

How can this be avoided? There is an obvious need to avoid aggravating loss which can be exacerbated by undignified situations and the wasting of the patient's time and energy with unnecessary investigations, appointments, and encounters with new staff at home or in hospital. It is particularly important not to induce cognitive deterioration by careless prescribing. There is more: clinicians need a more adequate understanding of the tasks of persons in the last decade (or two) of life, so that the work being undertaken by even the very frail elderly is given high priority in the minds of clinical decision-makers. Those in these last decades of life are very busy with demanding tasks to fulfil.

What are these tasks? One task is that of paying attention to all constitutive relationships, notably with persons, but also with place/things and so on – for example, personal projects which need to be brought to a conclusion, including estate planning, no matter how tiny the estate. These activities of closure do not at all preclude the making of plans for undertaking something new, although that is accompanied by a realistic recognition that the planter of seeds may not see or reap the harvest. Nor do they preclude a growing awareness that what one seeks to do and become will never be complete. This growing conviction, accompanied by an awareness of impending loss, can contribute to so-called anticipatory grief.

Closure activities may be very bound up with other persons. Significant relationships may need respect, fostering, and repair/restoration. The patterns are myriad and the realities, confidential. Staff have no right to an explanation. But time and energy may be critical and opportunities as well as privacy may need to be ensured somehow. (I once encountered a very elderly gentleman crying quietly in a hospital bed on a Saturday afternoon because complications of a necessary – but not urgent – biopsy the day before had prevented him from attending his granddaughter's wedding.)

A person living the last phase of life needs privacy both to explore the meaning of their situation and to perform these monumental tasks of preparing for the closing of their life. In health services characterised by teams (in both hospitals and especially in the community), extra care is needed to safeguard privacy. Concern for privacy should extend to spiritual privacy. There was, once, a vogue for developing a scale of spiritual health, of measuring even that most private of aspects of the self, the wellspring of personal life. The spiritual is the ground of person's sense of meaning and of their relations with persons, places, things, their remembered past, and also with all that is, namely transcendence. This is sacred ground. And no carer, even a pastoral carer, should seek to explore it or tread on it unless unshod and explicitly invited.

Exploration

Poets articulate some human truths in a way which gives the rest of us words to grasp. For example, T.S. Eliot:

> Old men ought to be explorers
> Here or there does not matter
> We must be still and still moving
> Into another intensity...[1]

What is this exploring all about?

85

There is new terrain to be negotiated. Symptoms such as weakness, pain, mobility issues, loss of energy may all be encountered, sometimes for the first time. Even the most sophisticated palliative medicine may not eradicate all of them.

New possibilities are glimpsed – new sources of joy and pain; new places and persons where beauty can be found; renewed appreciation of the kindness of strangers; new ideas, maybe to be connected with old insights; fresh framings of hope and a deepened respect for the rich fabric of human diversity. Indeed, there may be a fresh synthesis of the personal philosophy one fashions from the residues of past perspectives. Above all, there may be a new response to the haunting questions of Who and where am I now? Who is my neighbour? And what can I be for you? The particular becomes more and more precious as does the present moment.

There are new realities to be faced. One may be brought face to face with mortality by the death of a spouse or a friend or by one's own medical event. That may be a great shock and it calls not for retreat (geographical or chemical) but for a personal growth which can incorporate this human truth. Then again, there may be a new appreciation of the excellence of the skills of others and of one's utter dependence on persons who, hitherto, were only on the edges of one's awareness. These explorations yield human treasure and one is richer for the undertaking. In sum, there may be a more profound understanding of 'the whirling world of which one is a minute part'. (The philosopher Plotinus wrote on this in the third century.[2])

Caution is called for:

Where have I read that at the end, when life's surface upon surface, has become completely encrusted with experience, you know everything, the secret, the power, and the glory, why you were born, why you are dying, and how it all could have been different? You are wise. But the greatest wisdom, at that moment, is knowing that your wisdom is too late. You understand everything when there is no longer anything to understand.[3]

It may take both time and a sharp jolt to realise that living is in the exploring not in the finding. Clinicians may need to be more gentle with, and to, all.

Preparation for closing life, for the act of dying

The literature on the act of dying is influenced by larger perspectives on human life. The mediaeval *ars moriendi* and its successors reveal a view of human life itself as preparation for the world to come. But where this view does not prevail, other approaches to preparing for the end of one's life are mandated and clinicians need to have thought about such matters in order to care for very ill patients with sensitivity and integrity.

Each clinician and each patient will think about death in their own way. Clinicians and families alike may regard it simply as a therapeutic failure or error, a mode of thinking which disregards the complexity and mystery of human life and death. Or they may see it as the unthinkable having happened. Or as one ancient writer is said to have thought, death may be feared as though one were a gladiator waiting for the final blow. Then again, the end may be welcomed as a friend and a fitting conclusion to striving. Marxist philosopher Ernst Bloch wrote that dying is 'the master test of our journeyman years. It tests the value of our inner metaphysics...'[4]

It could be that, in most of us, all of these notions are present and mixed up with each other. All we can be sure of as clinicians or family members beside a bed at the moment of a person's death, is that now that person has passed away and is no longer there; what lies in that bed is truly the remains. (One finds more respect for the old terminology.)

There are other thoughts worth exploring.

The last movement of a symphony is a critical part of the whole, influenced profoundly by what has gone before, sometimes blending previously dissonant musical themes into a new synthesis. It is a work of art and such may be the last phase of life. It is a creative task to shape one's life according to whatever pattern one has in mind, recognising that it is not what happens but the responses to what happens which are the creative tools. One is responsible for what one becomes. Lisa Rosenbaum, national correspondent for the *New England Journal of Medicine*, wrote of empathic care for dying patients, concluding,

> The nature of prognostication means we will sometimes be wrong. And the nature of disease means we will often have no cure to offer. But the nature of hope requires a sort of empathy that is not about feeling what our patients feel, but instead about seeing in them what they can be.[5]

If we, clinicians and patients alike, recognise the last phase of life, especially but not only, when a person is close to dying, as a phase, not of deterioration, but one of artistry and becoming, then we are in step with a rich tradition of thought. We also have a chance to enrich ourselves and our hospitals and community at their roots – a truly radical enrichment.

6

After the Decade for Dying, What Now?

The previous chapter discussed what it was like to live in the decade of the dying – in Australia, the decade roughly between seventy-five and eighty-five years. But what if one has outlived that span of years, what then?

The earliest human records contain evidence that, among the core questions that deepen our wisdom in their exploration, are those of ageing, frailty and our own death. As the centuries went on, such wisdom became the province of philosophy and religion and, later still, great writers explored the terrain. All of these understandings of the temporary nature of the human condition become more arresting when one finds oneself there, in the place where they must be faced.

Erich Auerbach, German philologist and literary critic, gives us a pointer:

> We are constantly endeavouring to give meaning and order to our lives in the past, the present, and the future, to our surroundings, the world in which we live; with the result that our lives appear in our own conception as total entities – which to be sure are always changing, more or less radically, more or less rapidly, depending on the extent to which we are obliged, inclined, and able to assimilate the onrush of new experience.[1]

Giving meaning and order to our lives depends on how we assimilate the onrush of new experience. What happens in the future, from now on, and how I assimilate it – take it into my being – has a critical influence on my capacity to sustain a sense of my whole. But what do I know of my future? The only certainty is that I will come to the close of my life, that I will die. This is the known known. The rest is un-known. Almost certainly there will be distress – and even suffering as that sense of impending personal disintegration discussed in previous chapters – a sense of my centre not holding. Maybe the context will be so difficult that I will need to remember those who, in my own lifetime, remained capable of heroic morality in extreme conditions I cannot know or imagine.[2] I find it apposite to recall the words of the psychotherapist Victor Frankl, reflecting on the Nazi concentration camps: 'The last of human freedoms is to take an attitude in a given set of circumstances.'[3]

Maybe there will be not suffering but frailty, and maybe losses I have not foreseen, like loss of place, or of loved ones, of comfort, of cultural compatibility, of beauty in forms I cherish, of freedoms I value and of capacities (physical and intellectual) in which my security may rest.[4] Maybe the suddenness of the onrush of new experience will take me unawares. It is easy to lose heart, to be afraid. Afraid of much – but notably of frailty.

Frailty – the notion is worth a pause. The *Oxford English Dictionary* defines 'frail' as 'liable to be broken; easily destroyed. Weak. Easily overcome'. Frailty, then, is the liability to be crushed or to decay; perishableness; weakness. The nuance is unmistakeable and familiar with regard to material things, persons, and even concepts/perspectives which hitherto have seemed solid.

In fact, frailty is commonplace in the human condition, a facet of many lives. It is not restricted to old age but it is notable of the last phase of life and advanced age. The possibility of fragility and the press of contingency may induce dismay. It may invoke fear. It is hard to face frailty both in oneself and in another.

There is no place in frailty for the Tarzan complex, so pervasive in our times which glorify personal power and denigrate weakness. We have a distorted perception of both power and weakness – this is what I have called elsewhere 'the weak-strong dilemma'.[5] The oppression of the weak by the strong is the common core of travesties such as child abuse, elder abuse and domestic violence, as well as of war. And all this at a time when we need imagination to continually shape and reshape possibility in the midst of weakness. In some contexts, however, frailty is valued: consider the delicacy of porcelain, of a butterfly's wings, of a gossamer thread. Sometimes it is the stuff of poetry. Could the frail person ever be seen to be as beautiful and valuable as rare porcelain? What would it take to have such a seismic cultural shift? What would it cost society (or me) to look frailty in the face? Poets sometimes do.

> Frailty, now I have seen your face!
> fingered diaphanous hair yielding
> to breath gentle as child's sleep,
> and bending, I gaze at sweet, sweet eyes
> unseeing stars now, feet treading lightly
> in paths worn by ones remembered
> going before, going before…[6]

In fact, frailty, the propensity for being broken, like the fact of inevitable death, provides a frame in which one's basic notions can be tested, like an alloy is tested in fire. It is a complex, evocative, human reality worthy of careful exploration and this may just yield a new sense of possibility. For doctors, especially, and for others radically committed to the human good and human flourishing, it may yield a new understanding of responsibility. Clearly some notion of the human good and its concomitant, human flourishing, must be part of any serious reflection on frailty. For however these are conceived, frailty appears to endanger them.

So late old age has many recognisable features. But is this period essentially different from any other time of life? Really different? It has always been the case that we cannot determine the cards we are dealt in life but only how we play them. It has always been the case that the task of life is to become what we may truly be. We need wisdom but where is wisdom now to be found? It is sought, above all, in persons, but also in our roots and traditions, in art, in writings, in named disciplines, and in poetry. Recently, the literary critic Harold Bloom, after recovering from a near fatal illness and in a pensive mood, wrote, 'At the gates of death I have recited poems to myself, but not searched for an interlocutor to engage in dialectic.' For him, in his extremity, only the poetry he remembered nourished the mind and heart. In the same book, he suggested that 'We cannot all become philosophers, but we can follow the poets in their ancient quarrel with philosophy, which may be a way of life but whose study is death.' So Bloom sought, instead, the poetry which he remembered – for him, it was the poets, not the philosophers, who were the distillers of wisdom.

Even so, there is a place for philosophers. Maybe a resonance found there will occasionally carry us through our nights, when we most need light. The philosophy of Spinoza is one which offers insights useful for any stage of life, but poignantly relevant in very old age. The essence of his thought has been made accessible by the Australian philosopher, Genevieve Lloyd, amongst others.[8]

Conatus

One of Spinoza's central concepts if that of *conatus*, an old word best translated as 'the striving to continue in being'. Spinoza maintained that *conatus* is the essence, not only of human beings, but of all living beings and, indeed, of all things. We, the very elderly (and especially very elderly clinicians) have surely experienced this striving to continue in being and we have seen that striving in weak newborn babies and in patients emerging once more into life, after having come close to death. And, on others, we have witnessed the striving cease.

Conventional concepts like life force do not adequately express what is contained in the concept of *conatus*. Striving to continue in being implies, for me, as an ageing person, the impulse to continue being what I truly am – the concept contains a note of ontological authenticity. Does this mean that I strive to continue to live even at the increasing expense of others and that I never yield to the idea that the time has come to die? The American philosopher Margaret Battin (who I was privileged to meet) explored the possibility that there is a 'duty to die'.[9]

Ordinarily, striving to continue in being implies striving to continue to live as well as possible within whatever limits prevail. But someone who believes their continued being is costing others too dearly, may give rise to a duty to allow them to die. Indeed, there may well come a time when to continue in authentic being means to allow oneself to die, hopefully with dignity in the midst of good care. Dying may then be a time of completion, even celebration rather than a negation of life.[10]

The human person as part of nature

This notion is liberating! The recognition of our place in an interconnected web of 'all that is' issues in calm. Spinoza is a valuable contributor to the philosophical tradition which understands the relational constitution of the human being. He recognised that I, as a person, am essentially interconnected in time, and horizontally (so to speak) with other persons, that I am part of nature, part of the whole, a participant in its interconnectedness and so with responsibilities to care for the whole according to my capacity. Spinoza has been said to be the forerunner of deep ecology – for him, I am not above the rest of nature and I am who I am only in connectivity with other persons and with place. The relational view of a human person is central to Spinoza's thought. I am connected to what others have done, thought and been through what I know and remember as history and culture, including what others have hoped for and dreamt about. While he does not go further to conceive of relations as constitutive of person as I have rather boldly done, it would be interesting to discuss my view with scholars who are deeply immersed in his thought.

Freedom in contingency

There are ideas afoot that freedom is vested in autonomy. On reflection, though, one realises that freedom involves more than self-rule and the right to choose. Even in health care, choice is often glorified, not as a means, but as an end in itself, as the principal expression of autonomy.

There is a tendency for success to be measured by the pushing away of obstacles to individual desires – in other words, there is frustration in the face of what must be, of what philosophers call 'necessity'. These notions pervade the culture and require deep scrutiny. The freedom which education gives is not freedom of action, but freedom of thought and so educated, privileged, persons owe us that deep scrutiny. These questions are a backdrop to living in old age and may be critically at issue in the making of difficult clinical decisions.

In his famous essay 'On Liberty', written in 1859, the English philosopher J.S.Mill exalted the individualist idea of non-interference in one's life, by others, no matter how beneficent their motives:

> The principle is, that the sole end for which mankind is warranted, individually or collectively, in interfering with the liberty of action of any of their number is self-protection. That the only purpose for which power can be rightfully exercised over any member of a civilized community, against his will, is to prevent harm to others. His own good, either physical or moral, is not a sufficient warrant.

He went on,

> Each is the proper guardian of his own health, whether bodily, or mental or spiritual. Mankind are greater gainers by suffering each other to live as seems good to themselves, than by compelling each to live as seems good to the rest.

Clearly, the health of both individuals and the community both presupposes, and is expressed in, liberty. But how free are the decisions we make? How truly individual are our actions when viewed in the light of a relational concept of the person, with its implications for our understanding of human dignity, human suffering, and human complexity? The nature of persons in the human web is such that hardly any individual action fails to have social dimensions. Indeed, some actions said to be private and a matter for the individual are through and through social. These include how we are born, live, suffer, or how we love, hate, face frailty in our old age, or die.

Spinoza offered an alternative and far richer understanding. Genevieve Lloyd wrote,

> In Descartes' treatment of freedom, an inherently free will forces back ever further the limits of what must be accepted as beyond human control. The prevailing imagery is of border skirmishes... Spinoza offers instead a vision of freedom as the joyful acceptance of what must be... [F]reedom derives from the active engagement of the mind with necessity, an engagement that flows from the understanding of the truth.[11]

Freedom understood as the 'joyful acceptance of what must be' is not a recipe for passivity, nor fatalism, nor sheer stoicism. Spinoza's concept of *conatus* highlights the impulse inherent in all living things to continue in being and so is a long way from conventional determinism. Those of us not in a position to undertake a serious scholarly examination of his thought can still take from it an awareness the need to freely accept what must be, at the same time as we may be striving to relieve suffering and to enhance human flourishing.

It has often been said that Spinoza denied free will but this is to misunderstand his idea of freedom in contingency. Certainly, he insisted that the laws of nature cannot be broken, denying the possibility of miracles. Where Descartes conceived of freedom as residing in the will, Spinoza located it in our knowing. His view resonates with that of Frankl, quoted above: 'to take an attitude in a given set of circumstances' is a stance of the mind.

This is all a far cry from the prevailing view of autonomy as self-rule based on freedom of choice. It may be hard to accept but the highest expression of autonomy can be the yielding of control, a surrender in trust to the kindness of strangers. Cain's question, 'Am I my brother's keeper?' is still with us and the answer may be unwelcome. But there is a twist to it, for in a profound way, while being responsible selves, we are also a proximate other's keeper and we may need one day to turn and accept our keeping by another. In the sacred texts may be found the words 'Another may gird thee.'

The highest exercise of human knowing

Spinoza offers a way into a new humanism, a framework for our secular times – a humanism which takes into account the human awareness of a relation with all that is, however this be named and in whatever ritual, religious or otherwise, that awareness is expressed. (If ritual, as the anthropologist David Rappaport maintained, is a critical element in the evolution of humanity, understood not as the biologically evolved modern human but as humanity, then some ritual will often be involved in the awareness of all that is.[12])

In his day, Spinoza was scorned as an atheist. In my view, that was a misunderstanding which still affects even significant contemporary thinkers, for in fact he has a concept of God which is both rich and deep. For him, God is not essentially transcendent, separate from material reality, but is immanent in all reality. It is a view which could be labelled pantheist. But it could also be classed as panentheist, a term which suggests an immanent God overflowing and transcending the universe – both immanent and transcendent. (There are Christian theologians who rejoice in the notion of both transcendence and immanence, recognising an overflowing God as the beyond in the midst. Rabbis, too, traditionally recognise immanence while retaining a nuance redolent of overflow: 'God is the place of the world, but God's place is not the world.'[13] Outside the Judeo-Christian tradition, the emphasis on immanence is commonplace.) But the idea of God, whether or not wholly immanent, offers a grandeur for the mind to dwell upon. It is, as Wordsworth might say, a precious place for the 'mountings of the mind'.[14] Spinoza maintained that the highest activity of the human person is that of gazing on God.[15] At the very least, there is a focus here for the quiet or unquiet mind in the midst of, or at the close of, that striving (*conatus*) which is the essence of life. Such may be the heart of a radical humanism for our time. Meanwhile, thinkers continue to probe into the 'history of God'.[16]

Is Spinoza's idea that the highest human good is to gaze on God as the unity within all reality powerful enough to sustain one even when the centre seems not to be holding? Is a radical humanism centred on that thought able to sustain, not only patients, but also doctors in distress? Frailty may be feared by the very elderly even more than their approaching death. Can Spinoza illuminate the ambiguity of frailty as something both treasured and revered, yet feared? Maybe. For it could be that this understanding points the way to the recovery of integrity, that elusive wholeness which possible for each of us unique persons, even as we approach the close of life. Spiritual growth may be just this increasing clarity of awareness, and spiritual care (that controversial element in care) may simply be just the facilitation of that process (mainly by ensuring a clearing and utmost personal privacy).[17] The place is holy ground on which others should take off their shoes.

The thought world and the eternity of the mind

Spinoza anchors the mind in the body and much of his philosophy is in accord with contemporary neuroscience, which understands mind as a unique pattern of thought activity leaving its traces in the vast neuronal complexities of the brain.[18] But he also posited an eternal 'thought world' with which one's thoughts merge imperceptibly, to remain there forever. One's thinking is finished when one dies but one's thoughts are not lost. For better or worse, they endure as part of the whole, the eternal mind. To the mind of this non-philosopher, that rings true, and is a consoling thought.

Although we continually become aware of the limitations of our knowledge and understanding, there is a countermanding awareness of ageing clinicians that, taught by our failures, our successes and, above all, our patients, we have a store of human experience which may illuminate the questions, asked by scholarly disciplines, concerning the nature of the human person and our connections with all nature. We are singularly aware of the interconnectedness of the material web and the web of thought. We recognise with Spinoza the power of knowing, the power of being wholly aware. Spinoza may just be the guide for our times.[19]

Spinoza closes *The Ethics* with the following words:

An ignorant man, besides being agitated in many ways by external
causes, never possessing true contentment of mind also lives as it
were unaware of himself, God, and things, and as soon as he ceases
to be passive, ceases to be. On the other hand, the wise man, is
scarcely moved in spirit: he is aware of himself, of God, and things
by certain eternal necessity, he never ceases to be, but always pos-
sesses true contentment of mind. If the road I have shown to lead
to this is very difficult, it can yet be discovered. And clearly it must
be hard when it is so seldom found. For how could it be that if sal-
vation were close at hand and could be found without difficulty it
should be neglected by almost all? But all excellent things are as
difficult as they are rare.[20]

Is it the case that in very old age we need not only to be cared for
in our frailty, but above all, a clearing – a space in which we may grow
in being wholly aware?

Postscript

7

The Evolution of the Ecological Concept of a Person

We shall not cease from exploration
And the end of our exploring
Will be to arrive where we started
And know the place for the first time.
(T.S. Eliot, *Little Gidding*)

Genesis. In the late 1960s, when I was a newly fledged intern, it was rumoured that Aboriginal children were dying in Sydney hospitals.[1] Robert Black, of Sydney University's School of Public Health and Tropical Medicine, initiated a research project into the reasons for this. Recovering from a life-threatening illness, I was unable to do clinical work, so I assumed my alternative role as an academic and undertook an inquiry into aspects of the health of Aboriginal children in Sydney. This work became the basis of a doctorate thesis and its disturbing findings contributed to the formation of the Aboriginal Medical Service.[2]

At that time, the science of ecology was in the ascendant and living things were increasingly being understood in terms of their relationships with their environment – the concept of an ecology was ripe for expansion. In the course of my inquiry, I encountered the work of John Apley, a paediatrician, who wrote of a child as a 'unique ecological experiment'. The idea was powerful – and timely. I was able to fruitfully apply it to urban Aboriginal life so developing his ecological conception. It seemed clear to me that an Indigenous child was best understood if their personal history was taken into account, along with the other environmental features recognised by Apley.

I recognised, further, that this personal history stood like an edifice on a foundation called 'inheritance', which had two components – biological and cultural.[3] The bare bones of an ecological concept of the person were laid down and the resulting framework was to influence my subsequent work in Tasmania as a clinician, both as a researcher and as a medical educator.

Extension of the concept

In 1985, the nature of my clinical work changed. In Hobart, my main work had been in oncology. When I moved to the Royal Prince Alfred Hospital, a metropolitan teaching hospital of the University of Sydney and a significant centre for specialist training, my focus shifted to palliative medicine. At the request of clinical colleagues, I saw several thousands of patients in consultations over the next twenty-five years. Most were experiencing incurable illness and were in need, not only of symptom relief but also wise decisions and personal support. For most, this was achievable and their quality of life improved, even as they came close to death.

Our patients are our teachers – each one is a book to be read. It was the patients, their families, and the young trainee doctors who helped me realise that the ecological framework was of a closed system, in need of extension. The way out of that closure was the aspiration of the patient – hope. Hope is a vector leading out of that system. If one could understand what the patient most hoped for now and how they would formulate that, then one could gently assist them to settle on a reasonably realistic goal and so focus medical action and the action of one's team members far more effectively.

Later on, as the years passed and experience and reflection deepened, it seemed to me that the relations in my ecological conception should be thought of as interiorised, that they are not add-ons to an independently existing person but are actually *constitutive* of the person. Just as the filaments of a spider's web are the web, and the layers of an onion are the onion, so those relations do not merely characterise person but constitute them. This explains the pain of loss, whether it is loss of place, of persons, of significant things, of self-comfort (from pain, regret or bullying), of one's past (as memory fades) or loss of culture. There is a temporal dimension to each constitutive relation: all of them are in flux and subject to change. In teaching, the ecological view was now more often referred to as the 'relational' view of a person.

Each of the relations which together constitute the web of a person warrants further exploration.

Place

There are several senses of the word place, one of which is simply the geographical notion of land. This becomes personally significant when it is understood as 'my place' – a particularly strong notion with Indigenous Australians. Recent immigrants may have profoundly conflictual notions of place, Australian sites being just one of the places interiorised in a complex psyche.

Other persons

So profound are these relations that patients may become tense with anxiety about what is owed to another. If the pressure is too great, they may metaphorically go to pieces in the failed attempt to sustaining an interiorised relation with another.

In a dying person especially, part of the self may become as another person and intrapersonal dialogue may displace all else. The person may appear to be moving away from concern with both mundane affairs and other persons. He or she may then be like a boat casting off moorings, a distancing which needs to be understood and accepted for what it is, a final phase of growth. There is much about persons which is not measurable – or even comprehensible within our current conceptual framework.

Things

Those which count here are those which can be perceived to be embodied in a person and which can change as the self evolves.

The past

This is understood as that which is accessible through memory, including memories etched in the body, its cells, tissues, and organs, for these, like the memories in the mind, can bear traces of past experience. Memories can be heightened by some events which trigger reminiscence or they can be dulled by distractions or by drugs.

Culture

After noting how variously culture is defined, the anthropologist Clifford Geertz endorses the account of Max Weber, a view which resonates well with the ecological concept of person: 'Believing, with Max Weber, that man is an animal suspended in webs of significance he himself has spun, I take culture to be those webs.'[4]

There is another relationship which, during these years, emerged as constitutive of personhood. It is the phenomenon known as Marranism and it consists of identifiable players *within* an individual.[5] The term Marranism was first coined in sixteenth-century Spain where 'Marrano' was a derogatory label, one of its associations being with pigs. In that context it referred to Jews who had officially converted to Christianity, but had nevertheless persisted with traces of Jewish thought and practice. The philosopher Yovel has argued that this kind of multilayering has been significant in the evolution of the modern Western European person.[6] One can also expect to find it in immigrants.

If persons are constituted by their relations, they are necessarily always in flux, at the same time as there is continuity. A clinician working with the above ideas might fasten on the notion that it is the pattern of the complexus which persists throughout changes in the constitutive elements and their interactions. The strengthening and diminution of relations are inevitable over time. Hope – what the person most fundamentally desires – may also change shape over time. Changes come in a number of ways. Conversation within the self (the interior colloquium) is a powerful means of change. So is an experience of bonding, especially if wrought in fragile state. But despite all this, the pattern continues to be discernible. The patient holds it all together through *narrative*. I am, after all, my story.

Further extension: the spiritual dimension of care

There was more to come, but the final fundamental element in my schema was to be incubated for a decade or so. At issue were the notions of spiritual care and spiritual health, notions I had occasionally encountered at conferences and in conversations, not always in medical circles. I was uneasy about the relationship between spirituality and religion, because Australia is a secular nation where religion is understood to be a private matter. However, although we are individuals with personal opinions and our own cultural practice, doctors are also leaders who influence the culture of health services. In that culture, I realised, there was a need for clarity about what might be meant by spirit and the spiritual dimensions of care – the more so for those of us who do not see ourselves as very religious.

My approach to the question was via a notion of the whole. Each of us has some idea of the whole reality in which we are immersed, even though we are not usually aware of that dimension of our experience. There are different ways and times in which we are so aware: it may be that something takes us out of ourselves; we may have experienced ecstasy or had the 'oceanic' feelings discussed by Freud. We may experience this all that is when we gaze at the sea; walk in the wilderness; immerse ourselves in the wonders of a garden; delight in the look on a child's face; listen to music; make love; or become absorbed (we say) in art, or in tasks. And some of us also experience and express this same openness to the whole of reality in religious rituals.

Some name this whole, this all that is, God. Talk of God is pervasive, including in clinical contexts. (Jacob Needleman has recently written a book entitled *What is God?*) The God question is inescapable. We could accept that the 'all that is' be named God, if it is also acknowledged that there are many ways that God is conceived. There are those who understand God as transcendent, as creator, as sustainer and *carer* of all that is and there are those whose understanding is wholly of the immanent, of God as *present* within all that is. Where God is thought to be transcendent, petitionary prayer presupposes the possibility of the laws of the material universe being suspended. The alternative immanentist view would see prayer as mainly an expression of the awareness of 'all that is', and not as seeking miracles. In both cases, prayer is recognised as an aspect of humanness. There is a sense, then, in which the question 'Do you believe in God?' is irrelevant for doctors with an adequate concept of a person. If their understanding includes a notion of 'all that is', by whatever name, they may be a source of comfort and healing in a fragmented, distressed world. (In much later years, I have turned to Spinoza for further illumination of these issues.)

If the concept of God is somewhat fraught, so too are those of spirit and soul.[7] Clinical conversations usually avoid the topics, and yet they are at the core of humanness. Bypassing the philosophical discussions about immortality for the moment, it may be that we can find an understanding which enhances clinical practice, while avoiding the uneasiness and confusion surrounding these notions. I have suggested elsewhere that the spirit or soul could be seen as the principle of integration of a person, as whatever holds that complexity together. So understood, it would cease at death. The person is no longer there where the body lies; it has passed away. The folk expression is correct.

The conception developed here resonates with other perspectives on the human condition, notably those of human dignity and human suffering. Respect for the whole complexus is inherent in respect for human dignity,[8] while an operational definition of suffering is 'a sense of impending personal disintegration'.[9]

Torturers know how to induce distress and they do so deliberately, by violating the interiorised constitutive relations of a person. It is possible for well-meaning doctors to unwittingly induce distress, just by lack of awareness of the nature of the complexity of persons. We may simply know not what we do. It is time, then, to consider the implications of the relational view of a person for person-centred medicine.

Implications for medical practice and health services

Walt Whitman's words deserve to be posted on clinic walls: 'I am not contained between my hat and my boots.' (At least they should be brought to mind in every clinical encounter.) The patient embodies within him or herself a whole world of relations. While they may not have been explored, the attending clinician needs to be respectful of a continuing interior complexity. It is important not to assume, say, that no significant changes have developed since the last time appointment – in particular that there has not been a change in the configuration of hope. For all medical efforts need to focus on the personal goal, the locus of hope. This goal may be achievable or achievable only in part. Where it is not achievable at all the aim should be how to give comfort and/or how to refashion hope.

Clinical decisions and practice should involve this awareness of persons in all aspects of care: in history taking, diagnosis, therapy, communication, formulation of prognosis, rehabilitation, end of life care. How can this be done? Maybe some simple rules would help.

• Recognise the patient's narrative as the primary source of information concerning the patient as person and that it is *depersonalising* to reduce the patient's communication to data points'. Ask, for example, 'What happened to you to prompt you to come to see me/us now?'

• Clarify the shape of patient's hope/aspiration at this time, and the medically relevant obstacles to achieving this.

• Clarify the principal source of support for this patient at this time, and how this support is best made available. Is it a person and if so, how can they be contacted? Is it a place, maybe for reflection, for interior conversation, rest? Is it a treasured item? Perhaps a context which offers solitude is the immediate need.

• Respect the prioritisation of significant others as expressed by the patient.

• Respect the patient's culture, including their preferred modes of communication and traditional customs.

• Become aware of the patient's preferred way of being open to the whole (all-that-is) whether or not this is through ritual or understood as religious. This awareness would include avoiding clashes of medical appointments/investigations with significant events or customary activities.

• No matter how urgent the situation, gently ascertain if the patient is suffering in the sense of being about to go to pieces or unable to hold together. If they are, seek the cause or trigger. Then, try to not only comfort the patient, but modify planned procedures to minimise exposure to this trigger.

Implications for medical education

'Education' is etymologically related to the Latin words *educere* (to lead) and *educare* (to nourish). These two meanings are relevant to medical education for it involves the dimensions of both guidance and of nurturing.

In the course of medical education which continues throughout one's professional life, one should be 'led out' into new places, a result of increased information, knowledge, understanding and competence. One should also have been nourished and supported during this process within which one's own personal development would also have been occurring. Now, in clinical practice one encounters other persons in crisis, and, as Erikson taught us, crises facilitate personal growth. And while the medical student or doctor may encounter his or her own personal crises, these encounters with patients in crisis are significant educators.

It is the patient who displays the symptoms and signs of the diseases being studied and who is available to facilitate clinical research. Above all, though, it is the patient who can educate the clinician in all manner of aspects of humanness: in facing fear, managing anger, displaying unfailing integrity, behaving ethically as well as courageously, falling down and getting up again, forgiving and accepting forgiveness, caring for others or struggling with narcissism, grappling with loss, rejoicing in persons, place, things or memories, grieving for past failures yet grasping all the possibilities of the present, finding peace, accepting the approach of the end of life and even comforting the doctor trying to achieve the best possible outcome. Patients teach life skills to the doctor who will listen.

Conclusion

Kingsley Mortimer, a New Zealander professor of anatomy, once maintained that 'it is the task of medicine to emancipate man's interior splendour'.[10] One could elaborate further that it is the task of the enlightened clinician when seeking to relieve human suffering, to never lose hope in human possibility however dark the times, so to unmask that human grandeur.

In the end, it may be that the clinician owes gratitude for the privileged encounters with others in all their intrinsic complexity, diversity and uniqueness. For we not only encounter others – that is the stuff of life since we are all radically interlocked – but we get to walk beside them for a while and to be of assistance in times of extreme personal difficulty. We learn from them, not only how to treat disease but also how to recognise the world within ourselves, and we learn how to live and how to die.

Notes

Introduction

1. The German philosopher, Wilhelm Dilthey, amongst the first to make this distinction, developed criteria for the classification of an area of knowledge as a human science. (Dilthey, *Selected Works*, Vol. 1)
2. This address was a condensation of the ideas in Manderson, *Proximity, Levinas and the Soul of Law.*
3. Lickiss, 'The Human Experience of Illness'. 42–6.
4. Perhaps this world is alien only to the one educated professionals admit to inhabiting. Sometimes we attend the funeral of a mentor to find there an unexpected ritual. Is this just for the family or is it intrinsic to the life of our colleague we have known for some years? Surely he or she must have foreshadowed this even if they did not actually arrange it? How is it that they never spoke of it?
5. Huxley, ed., *The Humanist Frame.*

6. Watson, *A Terrible Beauty.*
7. Recent research has considered the role of patients' measures of outcomes of treatments: Black, 'Patient reported outcome measures', f266.
8. Watson, *The German Genius.*
9. Dworkin, *Justice for Hedgehogs.*
10. Needleman, 'The Perception of Mortality', 733–738.
11. Cassell, *The Nature of Suffering and the Goals of Medicine.*

Chapter 1

1. Sontag, *Illness as Metaphor*, 1.
2. Bircher, 'Towards a dynamic definition of health and disease', 335–341.
3. Exceptions are sudden, traumatic, deaths at an early age, such as those of young soldiers. Until very recently, more soldiers died of disease than of trauma and the same situation prevails in natural disasters. Illness, in other words, is mostly embedded in a life story; disease can

sometimes abruptly cut that story short.

4. Dilthey, *Selected works*, Vol. 1.
5. Thomasma et al., *Personhood and Health Care*.
6. A number of writers, among them Dewey, Thoreau and Conan Doyle, employ the metaphor 'the furniture of the mind'.
7. Taylor, *Sources of the Self*, 36.
8. Walt Whitman, 'Song of Myself', no. 7 in *Leaves of Grass*.
9. Quoted in Becker, *The Birth and Death of Meaning*, 43.
10. Ibid., 44.
11. Taylor, op. cit.; Siegel, *The Idea of the Self*.
12. Erikson, *The Life Cycle Completed* and *Identity and Life Cycle*.
13. Erikson, *Identity and Life Cycle*, 104.
14. Ibid., 104.
15. Mullan, 'Seasons of survival', 313:270–273.
16. Dow, 'The enduring seasons of survival', 511–6.
17. Little, 'Chronic illness', 201–202.
18. Corbin, et al., 'A nursing model for chronic illness management', 155–174.
19. Anderson, 'Living until we die', 213–225.
20. Dow, op.cit.
21. Loescher et al., 'Surviving adult cancers, Part 1', 411–432; 'Surviving adult cancers, Part 2', 517–524; Plowman et al., *Complications of Cancer Management*.
22. Nussbaum, *Upheavals of Thought*.
23. Gibson et al., 'Psychological issues in palliative care', 61–80; Steinhauser et al., 'Factors considered important', 2476–2482.
24. Turner et al., 'Dignity in dying', 7–13.
25. Lickiss, N. and M.G. Evans, unpublished observations, 1985.
26. Lee-Jones et al., 'Fear of cancer recurrence', 95–105.
27. Cicirelli, 'Personal meanings of death', 713–733. Penson et al., 'Fear of death', 160–9; Spiro et al., *Facing Death*.
28. Hockley, 'The concept of hope', 181–186.
29. Cutcliffe et al., 'The concept of hope in nursing', 42.
30. Nekolaichuk et al., 'On the nature of hope in palliative care', 36.
31. Morse et al., 'Delineating the concept of hope', 277–285.
32. Cassell, op. cit.
33. Turner, R.J., D.A. Lloyd, 'Lifetime traumas and mental health: the significance of cumulative adversity', *J. Health Social Behav.*, 1995: 36, 360–376.

34. Alter et al., 'Identification of PTSD in Cancer Survivors', 137–143.

35. Ironside et al., 'Experiencing chronic illness: creating new understandings', 171–183; Delmar et al., 'Achieving harmony with oneself', 204–212; Thorne et al., 'Two decades of insider research', 3–25.

36. World Health Organisation Expert Committee Report, *Cancer pain relief and palliative care*, Geneva: WHO, 1990.

Chapter 2

1. Lewis-Williams, T*he Mind in the Cave*; Mithen, *The Prehistory of Mind*.

2. *Iliad*, xxxiv, 502–6.

3. Zornberg, *The Beginning of Desire: Reflections on Genesis*.

4. Cassell, 'The nature of suffering', 639–645.

5. Russell, *The Autobiography*, Prologue.

6. Cherny, 'The problem of suffering', 306; Doyle et al., eds, *Oxford Textbook of Palliative Medicine*, 7–14; Daneault et al, eds, 'The Nature of Suffering', 7–11.

7. Needleman, 'The Perception of Mortality', 733–738.

8. Bloom, *Shakespeare*, xvii.

9. Shakespeare, *As You Like It*, Act II, scene ii.

10. Shakespeare, *Macbeth*, Act IV, Scene iii.

11. Antanovsky, *Unraveling the mystery of health*.

12. Taylor, *Sources of the Self*, 36.

13. Rehnsfeldt et al., 'The progression of suffering implies alleviated suffering', 264–272.

14. Morse, 'Towards a praxis theory of suffering', in *Adv Nursing Sci*, 47–59.

15. Rawlinson, 'The sense of suffering', 9–62.

16. Cassell, op. cit., 41–43.

17. Lickiss, 'On limits and liberty'.

18. Lickiss, 'The physician', 259–265; Lickiss, 'The human experience of illness', 42–46.

19. Christakis, *Death Foretold*; Glare et al., 'Predicting survival in patients with advanced disease', 1146–5.

20. Lickiss, 'On the Care of Our Aged: Privilege and Responsibility', in *Australian Rehabilitation Review*, 51–57.

21. Shaerer, 'Suffering of the doctor linked with death of patients', 27–37.

22. The work of Mary Vachon is noteworthy in this respect: Vachon, 'Reflections on Compassion, Suffering and Occupational Stress'.

23. Cole et al., 'The suffering of physicians', 1414–1415.

24. Alexander, 'Medical science under dictatorship', 40–47.
25. Ibid. 39–47.
26. These ideas resonate with those of Rawlinson, op. cit. See also Lickiss, 'On Human Dignity'.
27. Taboada, 'Human Dignity and the Ethics and Aesthetics of Pain and Suffering'.
28. Kingsley Mortimer quoted in Bishop, *Cancer Facts*, 81.

Chapter 3

1. The title of this paper comes from the Tennessee Williams play *The Streetcar Named Desire*, at the end of which, the promiscuous Blanche Dubois suffers a psychological breakdown and is led away to an asylum. 'Whoever you are,' she says to the doctor, 'I have always been dependent on the kindness of strangers.'
To avoid too much repetition with the ecological view of a person expounded in Part One of this book, this chapter is a very condensed version of the first Barbara Leroy Memorial Lecture, Annual Conference of Palliative Care Association, NSW, 2 November 2006.
2. Thornhill, *Making Australia: Exploring our National Conversation*.
3. David Hume, for example, maintained that sympathy (now called 'empathy') is the primary human response to another. (Hume, *A Treatise on Human Nature*)
4. Vanlaere et al., 'A normative approach to care ethics', 99–116.
5. Verkerk, 'Care ethics as a feminist perspective on bioethics', 65–79.
6. J. Tronto, *Moral Boundaries: A Political Argument for an Ethic of Care*, 1030.
7. Verkerk, 'Care ethics', 65–79.
8. Walt Whitman, 'Song of Myself'.
9. Taylor, *Sources of the Self*, 36.
10. Porter, *The Greatest Benefit to Mankind*, 245.
11. Manderson, 'Philosophical Basis of the Duty of Care'; Malpas, *Perspectives on Human Dignity*, 233.
12. Diedrich et al., 'Towards a Levinasian Care Ethic', 33–61.
13. Palliative medicine is not only that practised by palliative medicine specialists for a wide range of other doctors are involved the treatment of the patients concerned.
14. Committee on care at the end of life, *Approaching Death: Improving Care at the End of Life*.
15. Glare et al., 'Can we do better in end of life care?', 530–533.

16. Steinhauser at al., 'Factors considered important', 2476–82.
17. Ten Have et al., eds, *Bioethics in a European Perspective*.
18. Malpas, 'Human dignity and Human being'.
19. Enthoven, 'Cutting cost without cutting the quality of care', 1229–38.
20. Glare et al., 'Quality Assurance in Palliative Care', 572.
21. Lickiss, 'On the care of our aged', 51–57; Haynes, *Seeking the Centre*.
22. Alexander, 'Medicine under dictatorship', 40–47.
23. Forster, *A Passage to India*.
24. Haynes, op. cit.

Chapter 4

1. Inglefinger, former editor of the *New England Journal of Medicine*, is said to have been critical of his AMO when he was afflicted with ca oesophagus.
2. Enthoven, 'Cutting Cost', 1056.
3. For example, Christakis, *Death Foretold*.

Chapter 5

1. Eliot, *Four Quartets (East Coker)*.
2. Miles, *Plotinus on Body and Beauty*.

3. Eco, *Foucault's Pendulum*.
4. Bloch, *Man on His Own: Essays in the Philosophy of Religion*.
5. Rosenbaum, 'Falling together – empathic care for the dying', 587–590

Chapter 6

1. Auerbach, *Mimesis: The Representation of Reality in Western Literature*.
2. Todorov, *Facing the Extreme: Moral Life in the Concentration Camps*.
3. Frankl, *The Search for Meaning*.
4. Zander et al., *The Art of Possibility*.
5. Lickiss, 'Care of the Aged', 51–7.
6. Anonymous Australian poet, 'Response to a frail friend, bent low'.
7. Bloom, *Where Shall Wisdom be found?*
8. Lloyd, *Part of Nature: Self-Knowledge in Spinoza's ethics*; Lloyd, *Spinoza and the Ethics*.
9. Battin, 'Global Life Expectancies and the Duty to Die', 1–21.
10. Such a perspective on life at any adult age, but especially in old age, is in no way supportive of notions of suicide (however assisted) or euthanasia. It requires that the

patient (or person) be given relevant information about the cost to self and others of their continuing efforts to live or to be kept alive.

11. Lloyd, *Providence Lost*, 200 ff.
12. Rappaport, *Ritual and Religion in the Development of Humanity*.
13. The saying is attributed to R. Eliezer. See Plaut, ed., *The Torah: A Modern Commentary*, n. 38, 211, 1509; Yovel, *Spinoza and Other Heretics*, Vols 1 and 2.
14. Wordsworth, *The Prelude*: 'Traces of thought and the mountings of the mind/Come fast upon me'.
15. Lloyd, *Spinoza and the Ethics*, 109–131.
16. Armstrong, *A History of God*; Aslan, *God: A Human History of Religion*.
17. Lickiss, 'Palliative Care, Art and the Jewish Tradition'.
18. Damasio, *Looking for Spinoza*.
19. Lickiss, 'Can the Philosophy of Baruch Spinoza Enrich the Thinking of Doctors?'
20. Spinoza, *The Ethics*.

Chapter 7

1. The national referendum was held in 1967 and so concern about Aboriginal living conditions had been increasing throughout the 1960s.
2. Respect for the privacy of those interviewed meant that it was never published. (This was at my own request because there were no ethics committees in those days regulating such decisions.) There are, however, copies in some university libraries and some papers were published: Lickiss, 'Health Problems of Sydney Aboriginal children', 995–1000; 'Aboriginal children in Sydney: the socio–economic environment', 201–28; 'The Aboriginal people of Sydney with special reference to health of their children: a study in human ecology'.
3. With respect to the wider history of Sydney's Aboriginal people, my understanding was necessarily inadequate. At the time it was thought that Aboriginal people had been in the land now called Australia about 10,000 years – much less than the 50,000 or more now believed to be the case – but even so, considerably longer than the (then) less than 200 years of European settlement. However, it was just one year after the referendum which had resulted in Aboriginal citizenship

finally being recognised and Aboriginal thought and social patterns were, for the most part, ignored or at best treated as curiosities. Nor was the brutality of their experience after the arrival of the British common knowledge.

4. Geertz, *The Interpretation of Cultures*, 5.

5. Yovel, *The Other Within: The Marranos: Split Identity and Emerging Modernity*.

6. Ibid.

7. Among the vast literature on these subjects is one by the medical historian, Roy Porter: *Flesh in the Age of Reason: The Modern Foundations of Body and Soul.*

8. Lickiss, 'On Human Dignity', in Malpas et al., *Perspectives on Human Dignity*.

9. Ibid.

10. Reported in Bishop, *Cancer Facts*, 81.

Bibliography

Abbreviations

Adv Nursing Sci: *Advances in Nursing Science*
Ann Intern Med: *Annals of internal Medicine*
Annu Rev Nurs Res: *Annual Review of Nursing Research*
BMJ: until 2014, this was a shortening of *British Medical Journal*. *BMJ* is now the official title.
JAMA: *The Journal of the American Medical Association*
Med J Aust: *The Medical Journal of Australia*
New Eng J Med: *The New England Journal of Medicine*
Scand J Caring Sci: *Scandinavian Journal of Caring Sciences*

Alexander, L. 'Medical science under dictatorship'. *New Eng J Med* 24 (1949): 40–7.

Alter, C.L., Pelcovitz and Axelrod, A. 'Identification of PTSD in Cancer Survivors'. *Psychosomatics* 37 (1996): 137–143.

Anderson, H. 'Living until we die: reflections on the dying person's spiritual agenda'. *Anaesthesiology Clinics of North America* 42 (2006): 213–225.

Antanovsky, A. *Unraveling the mystery of health. How people manage stress and stay well.* San Francisco: Jossey-Bass Publishers, 1970.

Armstrong, Karen. *A History of God.* London: Heinemann, 1993.

Aslan, R. God: *A Human History of Religion.* London: Transworld, 2017.

Auerbach, E. *Mimesis: The Representation of Reality in Western Literature (1942–45),* translated by W.R. Trask. Princeton: Princeton University Press, 2003.

Barbato, M.P. 'Death is a Journey to be Undertaken'. *Med J Aust* 168, no. 6 (1998): 296–7.

Battin, Margaret B. 'Global Life Expectancies and the Duty to Die', in *Is There a Duty to Die?: Biomedical Ethics Reviews*, ed. James M. Humber and Robert F. Almeder (Atlanta, Georgia State University), 1–21.

Becker, Ernst. *The Birth and Death of Meaning: An Interdisciplinary Perspective on the Problem of Man*. Harmondsworth: Penguin Books, 2nd edition, 1971.

Bishop, James. *Cancer Facts*. CRC Publishers, 1999.

Bircher, Johannes. 'Towards a dynamic definition of health and disease'. *Medicine, Health Care and Philosophy* 8, no. 3 (2005):335–341: (https://doi.org/10.1007/s11019-005-0538-y.

Black, Nick. 'Patient reported outcome measures could help transform healthcare'. *BMJ* 346 (2013): f266.

Bloch, Ernst. *Man on his Own: Essays in the Philosophy of Religion,* edited by Jürgen Moltmann and Reiner Strunk, translated by E. B. Ashton. New York: Herder & Herder, 1970.

Bloom, Harold. *Shakespeare: The Invention of the Human*. New York: Riverhead Books, 1998.

—. *Where Shall Wisdom be found?* New York: Riverhead Books, 2005.

Cassell, Eric J. 'The goal of medicine the relief of suffering'. *New Eng J. Med* 306 (1982): 639–645.

—. *The Nature of Suffering and the Goals of Medicine*. Oxford: Oxford University Press, 2009.

Cherny, N. 'The problem of suffering'. *Oxford Textbook of Palliative Medicine,* 3rd edition. Oxford:Oxford University Press (2003).

Cicirelli, V.G. 'Personal meanings of death'. *Death Studies* 22 (1998): 713–733.

Christakis, N.A.. *Death Foretold: Prophecy and Prognosis in Medical Care*. Chicago: University of Chicago, 1999.

Committee on care at the end of life. *Approaching Death: Improving Care at the End of Life*. Washington DC: Institute of Medicine, National Academy Press, 1997.

Cole, T.R. and N. Carlin. 'The suffering of physicians'. *The Lancet 374* (2009): 1414–1415.

Corbin, J.M. and A. Strauss. 'A nursing model for chronic illness management based on the Trajectory Framework'. *Scholarly Inquiry for Nursing Practice 5* (1991): 155–174.

Cutcliffe, J.R and K. Herth. 'The concept of hope in nursing 1: Its origins, background and nature'. *British Journal of Nursing* 11 (2002): 832–840.

Damasio, Antonio. *Looking for Spinoza*. London: Vintage, 2004.

Daneault, S., V. Lussier, S. Mongeau et al. 'The Nature of Suffering and its Relief in the terminally ill: a qualitative study'. *Journal of Palliative Care* 20, no. 1 (2004): 7–11.

Delmar, C., T. Bõje, D. Dylmer et al. 'Achieving harmony with oneself: life with a chronic illness'. *Scandinavian Journal of Caring Science* 2005 (19): 204–212.

Diedrich, W.W., R. Burggraeve and C. Gastmans. 'Towards a Levinasian Care Ethic: A Dialogue between the thoughts of Joan Tronto and Emmaqnuel Levinas'. *Ethical Perspectives: Journal of the European Ethics Network* 13, no. 1 (2003): 33–61.

Dilthey, Wilhelm. *Selected works, Vol. 1: Introduction to the human sciences,* edited and and translated by R.A. Makkreel et al. Princeton, NJ: Princeton University Press (1985).

Dow, K.H. 'The enduring seasons of survival'. *Oncology Nursing Forum 17* (1990): 511–6.

Doyle, D., G.W. Hanks, N. Cherny and K. Calman, eds. *Oxford Textbook of Palliative Medicine,* 3rd edition.

Dworkin, Ronald. *Justice for Hedgehogs*. Harvard: Harvard University Press (2011).

Eco, Umberto. *Foucault's Pendulum,* translated by William Weaver. London: Seeker and Warburg,1989.

Eliot,T.S. *Four Quartets (East Coker).*

Enthoven, A.C. 'Cutting cost without cutting the quality of care'. *N Eng J Med* 298 (1978):1229–38.

Erikson, Erik H. *The Life Cycle Completed: A Review.* New York: Norton, 1982.

—. *Identity and Life Cycle, Psychological Issues Monograph.* New York: International Universities Press, 1969.

Feinstein, A.R. 'Clinical Judgement Revisited: The Dispaptraction of Quantitative Models'. *Ann Intern Med* 120 (1994): 799–805.

Forster, E.M. *A Passage to India. London:* Edward Arnold, 1924.

Frankl, Victor. *The Search for Meaning.* Boston: Beacon Press, 1959.

Geertz, Clifford. *The Interpretation of Cultures.* Basic Books. 1973.

Gibson, C.A., W. Lichtenthal, A. Berg, W. Breitbart. 'Psychological issues in palliative care'. *Anaethesiology Clinics of North America* 24 (2006): 61–80.

Glare, P., C. Sinclair, M. Dowing, P. Stone, M. Maltoni, A. Vigano. 'Predicting survival in patients with advanced disease'. *European Journal of Cancer 44,* no. 8 (2008): 1146–5

Glare, P.A., K. Virik. 'Can we do better in end of life care? The mixed management model and palliative care'. *Med J Aust 175* (2001): 530–533.

Glare, P.A., J.N. Lickiss. 'Quality Assurance in Palliative Care' (letter). *Med J Aust* (1992): 157:572.

Haynes, R. *Seeking the Centre: The Australian Desert in Literature, Art and Film.* Cambridge: Cambridge University, 1998.

Hockley, J. 'The concept of hope and the will to live'. *Palliative Medicine* 7 (1993) (181–186).

Huxley, Sir Julian, ed. *The Humanist Frame.* London: Allen & Unwin, 1961.

Hume, David. *A Treatise on Human Nature* (many editions).

Ironside, P.M., M. Schekel, C. Wessels et al. 'Experiencing chronic illness: creating new understandings'. *Qualitative Health Research* 13 (2003): 171–183.

Lee-Jones, C., G. Humphris, R. Dixon et al. 'Fear of cancer recurrence – a literature review and proposed cognitive formulation to explain exacerbation of recurrence fears'. *Psycho-oncology* 6 *(*1997): 95–105.

Lickiss, J. Norelle. 'Health Problems of Sydney Aboriginal children'. *Med. J. Aust* 1971: 995–1000: https://www.sciencedirect.com/science/article/pii/0037785675900037.

—. 'Aboriginal children in Sydney: the socio–economic environment'. *Oceania 41*, no. 2 (1971): 201–28.

—. 'On limits and liberty: an exploration'. Inaugural Professorial Lecture, Hobart. *University of Tasmania Occasional Paper no. 8*, 1977.

—. 'On the Care of Our Aged: Privilege and Responsibility'. *Australian Rehabilitation Review 2*, no. 6 (1982): 51–57.

—. 'On Human Dignity', in *Perspectives on Human Dignity: a Conversation*, edited by Norelle Lickiss and Jeff Malpas. Springer, 2007.

—. 'The Human Experience of Illness', in *Palliative Medicine*, edited by Declan Walsh, 42–6. Philadelphia: Saunders Elsevier, 2009.

—. 'The physician', in *Palliative Medicine*, edited by David Walsh, 259–265. Philadelphia: Saunders Elsevier, 2009.

—. *The Aboriginal people of Sydney with special reference to health of their children: a study in human ecology*. Sydney: Department of Tropical Medicine, School of Public Health and Tropical Medicine, 1971. mimeographed.

—. 'Palliative Care, Art and the Jewish Tradition'. Unpublished lecture, 2017.

Little, M. 'Chronic illness and the experience of surviving cancer'. *Internal Medicine Journal 34* (2004): 201 –202.

Loescher, L.J., D. Welch-McCaffrey, S. Leigh, B. Hoffman, F.L. Meyskens. 'Surviving adult cancers, Part 1: Physiologic effects'. *Annals of Internal Medicine 111* (1989): 411–432.

Lloyd G. *Part of Nature: Self-Knowledge in Spinoza's Ethics*. London: Cornell University Press, 1994.

—. *Spinoza and the Ethics*. London: Routledge, London. 1996.

—. *Providence Lost*. Cambridge Mass.: Harvard University Press, 2008, 200 ff.

Malpas, Jeff. 'Human Dignity and Human Being', in *Perspectives on Human Suffering*, edited by Jeff Malpas and Norelle Lickiss. Springer, 2012.

Manderson, Desmond. *Proximity, Levinas and the Soul of Law*. Montreal: Mc Gill-Queens University Press, 2007.

—. 'Philosophical Basis of the Duty of Care'. Annual symposium, Sydney Institute of Palliative Medicine (2001). Unpublished.

Meier, D.E., A.L. Back, R.S. Morrison. 'The inner life of physicians and the care of the seriously ill'. *JAMA 286*, no. 3 (2001), 3007–3014: doi:10.1001/jama.286.23.3007.

Miles, Margaret. *Plotinus on Body and Beauty.* Oxford: Blackwell, 1999.

Morse, J.M., B. Doberneck. 'Delineating the concept of hope'. *Sigma Theta Tau International* 27 (1995): 277–285.

Morse, J.M. 'Towards a praxis theory of suffering'. *Adv Nursing Sci* 24, (2001): 47–59.

Mullan, F. 'Seasons of survival: reflections of a physician with cancer'. *New Eng J Med 313* (1985): 270–273.

Needleman, Jacob. 'The Perception of Mortality'. *Annals of the New York Academy of Science 164*, no. 3 (1969): 733–738.

Nekolaichuk, C.L., E. Bruera, 'On the nature of hope in palliative care'. *Journal of Palliative Care 14* (1998): 36.

Nussbaum, Martha. *Upheavals of Thought: The Intelligence of Emotions.* Cambridge: Cambridge University Press, 2002.

Penson, R.T., R.A. Partridge, M.A. Shah et al. 'Fear of death'. *Oncologist 10* (2005): 160–9.

Plowman, P.N., T.J. McEwain, A.T. Meadows. *Complications of Cancer Management.* Oxford: Butterworth-Heinemann, 1991.

Porter, Roy: *Flesh in the Age of Reason: The Modern Foundations of Body and Soul.* W.W. Norton Company, 2005.

—. *The Greatest Benefit to Mankind. A Medical history of humanity from Antiquity to the Present.* London: Harper Collins, 2017.

Rappaport, R.A. *Ritual and Religion in the Development of Humanity.* Cambridge: Cambridge University Press, 1999.

Rawlinson, M. 'The sense of suffering'. *The Journal of Medicine and Philosophy 11* (1986): 39–62.

Rehnsfeldt, A., K. Eriksson. 'The progression of suffering implies alleviated suffering'. *Scand J Caring Sci* 18 (2004): 264–272.

Rosenbaum, Lisa. 'Falling together – empathic care for the dying'. *NEJM 6* (2016): 374:6; 587–590.

Russell, Bertrand. *The Autobiography of Bertrand Russell: 1872–1914.* London: George Allen and Unwin.

Shaerer, R. 'Suffering of the doctor linked with death of patients'. *Palliative Medicine* 7 (1993): 27–37.

Siegel, J. *The Idea of the Self: Thought and Experience in Western Europe since the Seventeenth Century.* Cambridge: Cambridge University Press, 2005.

Sontag, Susan. *Illness as Metaphor.* New York: Vintage Books, 1979.

Spinoza, Baruch. *The Ethics* (1675). translated by A. Boyle and G.H.R. Parkinson. London: Dent, 1989.

Spiro, H.M., M.G. McCrea-Curnen, L. Palmer Wandel, eds, *Facing Death: Where Culture, Religion, and Medicine Meet.* New Haven: Yale University Press, 1996.

Steinhauser, K.E., N.A. Christakis, E.C. Clipp et al. 'Factors considered important at the end of life by patients, family, physicians, and other care providers'. *JAMA* 84 (2002):2476–2482.

Taylor, Charles. *Sources of the Self: the Making of Modern Identity.* Cambridge: Harvard University Press, 1989.

Ten Have, H.A., B. Gordijn, eds. Dordrecht: Kluwer Academic Publishers, 2001.

Thomasma, D.C., D.N. Weisstub, C. Hervé et al., eds. *Personhood and Health Care.* Dordrecht: Kluwer, 2001.

Thorne, S.E., B.L. Paterson. 'Two decades of insider research: what we know and don't know about chronic illness experience'. *Annu Rev Nurs Res* 8 (2000).

Thornhill, John. *Making Australia: Exploring our National Conversation.* Newtown: Millennium Books, 1992.

Todorov, T. *Facing the Extreme: Moral Life in the Concentration Camps*, translated by A. Denner and A. Pollack. London: Weidenfeld & Nicholson, 1999.

Tolstoy, Leon. 'Non Acting'. *Recollections and Essays*, translated by A. Maude. London: Oxford University Press: 1937.

Tronto, J. *Moral Boundaries: A Political Argument for an Ethic of Care.* London and New York: Routledge, 1994.

Turner, K., R. Chye, G. Aggarwal et al. 'Dignity in dying: a preliminary study of patients in the last three days of life'. *Journal of Palliative Care 12* (1996).

Turner, R.J., D.A. Lloyd. 'Lifetime traumas and mental health: the significance of cumulative adversity'. *Journal of Health and Social Behaviour* 36 (1995): 360–376.

Vachon, Mary L.S. 'Reflections on Compassion, Suffering and Occupational Stress', in Jeff Malpas and Norelle Lickiss, eds. *Perspectives on Human Suffering*. Springer, 2012.

Vanlaere, L. and C. Gastmans. 'A normative approach to care ethics : the contribution of the Louvain tradition of personalism', in *New Pathways to European Bioethics,* et al., edited by C. Gastman. Antwerp and Oxford: Intersentia; 2007, 99–116.

Verkerk, M. 'Care ethics as a feminist perspective on bioethics', in *New Pathways to European Bioethics*, et al., edited by C. Gastman. Antwerp and Oxford: Intersentia; 2007, 65–79.

Watson, Peter. *A Terrible Beauty: The People and Ideas That Shaped the Modern Mind: A History.* Melbourne: Phoenix Press, 2001.

—. *The German Genius: Europe's Third Renaissance, the Second Scientific Revolution and the Twentieth Century.* London: Simon and Schuster, 2010.

World Health Organisation Expert Committee Report. *Cancer pain relief and palliative care.* Geneva:WHO, 1990.

Yovel, Y. *The Other Within: The Marranos: Split Identity and Emerging Modernity.* Princeton: Princeton University Press, 2009.

—. *Spinoza and Other Heretics*, Vols 1 and 2. Princeton: Princeton University Press, 1992.

Zander, R.S. and B. Zander. *The Art of Possibility.* Boston: Harvard Business Press, 2000.

Zornberg, Avivah Gottlieb. *The Beginning of Desire: Reflections on Genesis.* New York: Doubleday, 1995.